THE DANIEL FAST COOKBOOK

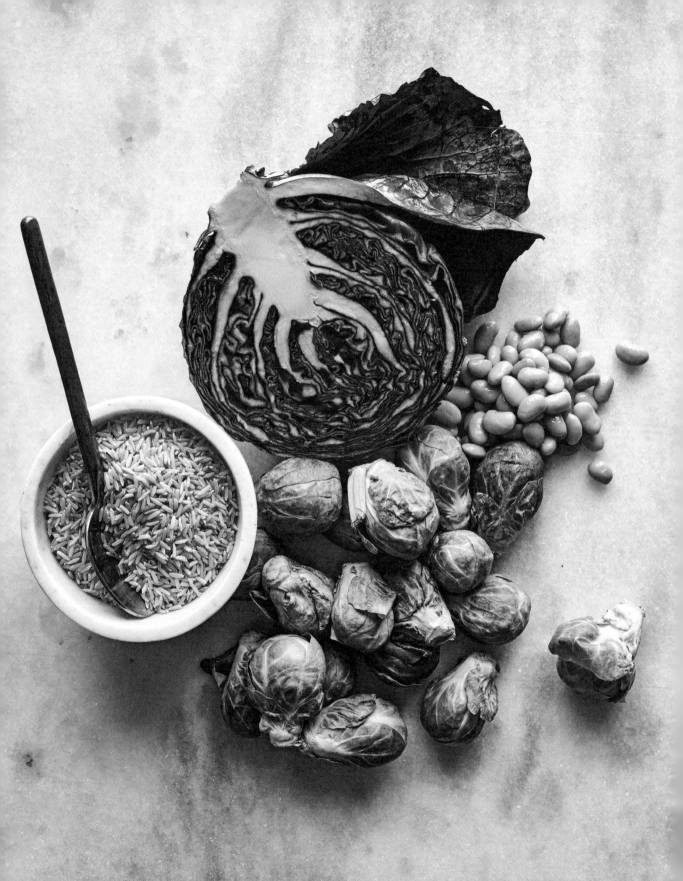

THE DANIEL FAST COOKBOOK

MEAL PLANS + RECIPES
to Bring You Closer to God

Cindy Anschutz

Photography by Emulsion Studio

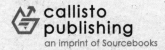
callisto publishing
an imprint of Sourcebooks

Published by Callisto Publishing LLC C/O Sourcebooks LLC

P.O. Box 4410, Naperville, Illinois 60567-4410

(630) 961-3900

callistopublishing.com

Printed and Bound In China

OGP 17

To my very dear friends,

Mike and Angela.

Without you, I wouldn't have met

Jesus or know His peace.

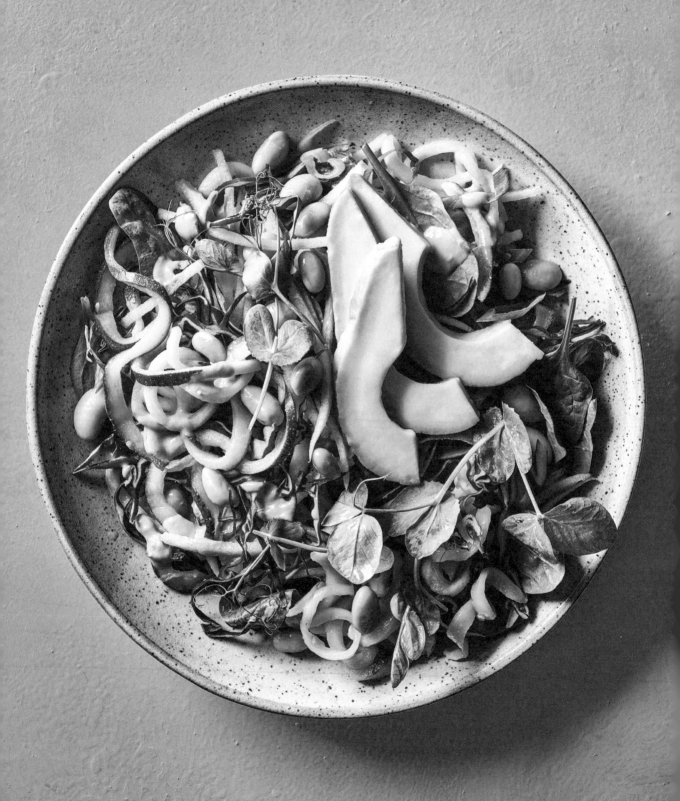

Contents

Foreword

You hold in your hand more than a cookbook. You're holding an invitation to share a meal with the Creator of the world. Throughout the Old and New Testaments, food appears again and again in the pages of scripture. From Eve eating of the tree to the promise of supper in heaven, the Bible has a lot to say about food. Our view of food has a lot to do with our view of the Creator. And Cindy Anschutz invites us to enjoy a meal that will sharpen our view of God and bring us closer to Him.

Cindy is not only a talented chef and writer, she is also a vibrant part of the local church. She serves and influences others through her craft of cooking and her calling as a follower of Jesus. Just as Jesus used the table and meal to connect with others, Cindy is inviting us to connect with Him through these meals. As you fall in love with these recipes, I trust you will fall more in love with the scriptures and with God Himself.

The invitation is open to all who would answer. Go ahead and set the table. Prepare the meal and open your heart to see God more clearly.

Pastor Dave Simiele
Campus Pastor
Christ Fellowship Church

Introduction

Before I became a believer, I didn't think God loved me. As a divorced woman with two kids, it had been impressed upon me that I didn't belong to the "church crowd." In 2015, my husband and I moved to South Florida, and in all honesty, finding a church was not on my agenda. However, I decided to attend church for Christmas and Easter—yes, I was a "Creaster"—even though I had been led to feel I didn't belong.

Then I was introduced to one of my now-close friends during a networking event. Our conversation moved to Jesus and quickly grew more serious. I told my friend and her husband that I didn't believe God loved me. Soon after, they invited me to their church. We sat in the back, and I honestly wasn't sure what to think of it, but something within me felt moved and renewed. Finally, I felt like I might be accepted in the church. Maybe God loved me after all. I wasn't exactly sure yet, but I kept coming back each week on my own, still taking it all in from the back row.

After a few months, I began attending a four-week seminar on God and our church. There I met a pastor and immediately started getting involved in service. It has been an amazing journey becoming part of a wonderful church and knowing that God does in fact love me!

It was at this wonderful church that I first learned about and began participating in the Daniel Fast, a partial fast based on the one described in the book of

Daniel. This fast is an opportunity to pray and worship while consuming what the Lord has naturally provided, pressing into Him as your sustainer in the moments when this fast is most difficult. Use a journal to keep track of what you eat or drink, and also write down the prayers you have in those quiet moments with the Lord. Personally, I always start my journal with my reasons for dedicating this time to the Daniel Fast.

Above all: *surrender*. There's no greater experience than surrendering our lives to the Lord. As believers, we're not called upon to be comfortable, and submitting to that reality is never easy. But by setting out on the Daniel Fast, you're making a commitment to the Lord, and that is always an inspiring venture. It is truly humbling to watch another believer step out in faith knowing the Lord will act. I pray that He will move mightily in you, revealing the "hope to which he has called you" and the "immeasurable greatness of his power" throughout this journey (Ephesians 1:19, ESV).

I hope this cookbook and devotional will help you surrender to the Lord with the Daniel Fast, whether you're doing the simple 10-day fast or the flexible 21-day fast. I also hope you build confidence in yourself knowing that God loves you and is always waiting to listen to your prayers. I'm thankful you've decided to go on this journey with me as we all draw closer to God with the biblical practice of fasting.

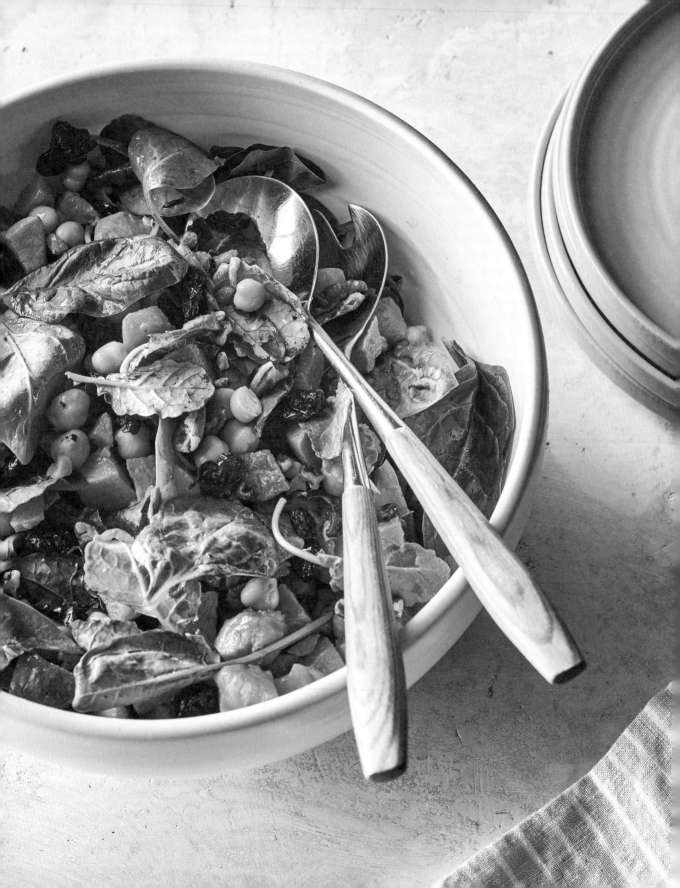

PART I

THE DANIEL FAST

1

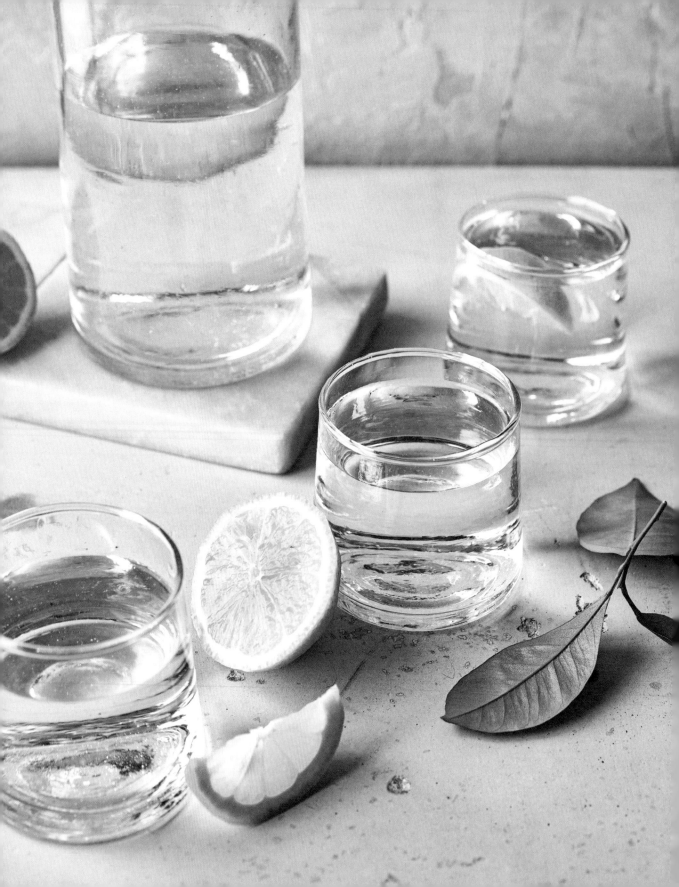

All About the Daniel Fast

Whether you've done the Daniel Fast before or are participating for the first time, we're all in this together! In this chapter, we'll go over the basics of the Daniel Fast: what it is, where in the Bible it comes from, and how the Lord can use this time as a radical period of growth in your faith journey.

WHAT IS THE DANIEL FAST?

Although fasting is a spiritual discipline that has virtually disappeared from culture today, it can hold some of the most profound experiences with the Creator for any believer. As we look into seeking a greater understanding of the Daniel Fast, we must understand that its purpose is greater than any weight-loss trend or fad diet that society has created. Fasting isn't for those seeking a shallow, comfortable faith. In his book *Habits of Grace*, David Mathis says that fasting is "for those who want more of God's grace. For those who feel truly desperate for God." As we dive further into what this looks like for us, let's make this our anthem in celebrating the Lord's provision and sustaining grace in our lives.

So, what is the Daniel Fast? Simply stated, it's a partial fast modeled after the fasts undertaken by Daniel in the Bible. Based on Daniel 1 and Daniel 10, the Daniel Fast relies on a plant-based diet, which removes all animal products and uses whole grains, vegetables, and water as your main sources of provision. Why would Daniel subject himself to that?

Well, during this time, the land of Judah had been overtaken by King Nebuchadnezzar of the Babylonian Empire. The holy temple in Jerusalem had been destroyed, and the Jews had been exiled to Babylon. Looking through the Old Testament, we find that this period of time was a fulfillment of the prophecies of Jeremiah, Ezra, and Ezekiel, among others. This exile was actually a punishment from God because of the disobedience of the people. But God said, "When seventy years are completed for Babylon . . . I will come to you and fulfill my good promise to bring you back to this place. For I know the plans I have for you . . . plans to prosper you and not to harm you, plans to give you hope and a future" (Jeremiah 29:10–11). After 70 years, God would indeed allow Persia to conquer Babylon, and the Jews would return to Jerusalem and rebuild the temple. He used a season of hardship to fulfill the promise He made to His people.

But none of that has happened yet in the book of Daniel. In chapter 1, we find Daniel and other promising young Jewish men being held in King Nebuchadnezzar's court. The intention was to assimilate them into Babylonian culture and train them to serve the empire. However, throughout this book, we find Daniel—whose name means "God is my judge"—consistently refusing to subject himself to the king's requests and remaining loyal to God. Daniel trusted that no matter what the rulers of this world did to him, the Lord would show him victory.

One of the many ways he did that was to not eat the food offered to him by the Babylonian court, which did not follow kosher dietary laws and was thus considered impure. There are actually two separate passages describing this partial fast; one is in Daniel 1 and one is in Daniel 10. Let's take a closer look at these verses and how Daniel used these restrictions to exalt the Lord and prove His intended deliverance for His people.

The Fast in Daniel 1

We find Daniel's first fasting experience in Daniel 1:8–21. Daniel and other young Jewish men (including Shadrach, Meshach, and Abednego, whom God would later protect in the fiery furnace) were chosen by the king's "chief official," Ashpenaz, to learn the ways of the Babylonians and serve in the royal court. Their menu was that of the king, yet Daniel and his friends resolved to resist defiling themselves by eating royal food or wine, which didn't follow the God-given dietary laws they observed.

When they requested only "vegetables to eat and water to drink," Ashpenaz hesitated. If they performed badly or looked unhealthy due to hunger, he himself would be punished. But Daniel challenged the steward to let them observe this partial fast for 10 days and judge what would take place after this period of time. And what an amazing testimony there was! "At the end of the ten days they looked healthier and better nourished than any of the young men who ate the royal food" (Daniel 1:15).

The Lord didn't just sustain them, He provided them with abundant physical health because of their desire to serve Him. And because they did so, the Lord had compassion and showed favor on Daniel and his friends. He gave them "knowledge and understanding of all kinds of literature and learning" and gave Daniel the ability to "understand visions and dreams" (Daniel 1:17). "In every matter of wisdom and understanding . . . [the king] found them ten times better than all the magicians and enchanters in his whole kingdom" (Daniel 1:20).

The Fast in Daniel 10

Although it was undertaken in different circumstances from the first, the fast in Daniel 10 was no less miraculous than the one in Daniel 1. In chapter 9, it was revealed to Daniel that there would be a time of great conflict (remember, in chapter 1, he was granted the ability to interpret visions and dreams). In Daniel 10:1–3, we see that these revelations from the Lord sent Daniel into mourning, and he ate no meat, wine, or "choice food" for three weeks.

As we read further into this passage, we see how the Lord answered Daniel because of his reverence and obedience: "Do not be afraid, Daniel. Since the first day that you set your mind to gain understanding and to humble yourself before your God, your words were heard, and I have come in response to them" (Daniel 10:12). Through Daniel's time of fasting, God brought revelation.

THE RULES

Because it's based on a few short Bible verses, there is no universally accepted set of criteria for the Daniel Fast. But for the purposes of this book, the Daniel Fast consists of following a plant-based diet as well as praying to God and gaining a closer relationship with him. Based on what the Bible says, the Daniel Fast means:

- "vegetables to eat and water to drink" (Daniel 1:12)

- "no choice food; no meat or wine" (Daniel 10:3)

Does that really mean you can only eat vegetables and drink water? Not quite.

First, the Hebrew word used means anything grown from seed, not just vegetables. So fruits, nuts, whole grains, and other foods that come from plants are totally acceptable. However, animal products like meat, dairy, and eggs are not.

Second, while some argue that you should drink only water—ideally distilled or purified water—others say that you should just avoid alcohol and caffeine. Ultimately, it's up to you. I think it's okay to drink fruit or vegetable juices or smoothies if you make them yourself at home. If you feel you need that one cup of coffee a day, be up-front about it, write it in your journal, and pray! After all, the Daniel Fast is more about prayer than about food. I think God would rather have you be honest in the beginning than fail and become discouraged.

Third, most people doing the Daniel Fast take "no choice food" as a cue to avoid sweets, processed snacks, and other "junk" foods. For many of us, gluten has become a choice food, so all the recipes in this book will be gluten-free. However, some people who do the Daniel Fast still eat wheat. Just make sure you avoid processed forms of wheat such as store-bought bread, bread products, and white flour. Instead, stick to whole-wheat flour.

Foods to...

EAT	AVOID	OPTIONAL
Fruits and vegetables (fresh, frozen, dried, or canned with no sugar added)	Meat	Fruit/vegetable juices or smoothies (homemade)
Whole grains (brown rice, barley, quinoa, farro, etc.)	Poultry	Decaffeinated coffee
	Fish	Herbal tea
Herbs and spices (fresh or dried)	Dairy (milk, butter, cheese, etc.)	Whole-wheat flour
Legumes (lentils, peas, beans, etc., dried or canned)	Eggs	
	Honey	
Nuts and seeds (peanuts, almonds, cashews, sunflower seeds, pumpkin seeds, etc.)	Bread and bread products (pasta, bagels, etc.)	
All-natural peanut butter (and other nut butters)	Candy, gum, sweets, and desserts	
Plant-based oils (olive, avocado, coconut, etc.)	Chips and other salty snacks	
Nondairy milks, unprocessed (coconut milk) or homemade (soy, almond, etc.)	Solid fats (even if they're plant-based, like margarine)	
Tofu	Sugar	
Water (preferably distilled or purified)	Salt with additives (iodized salt)	
Salt without additives (sea salt, Himalayan salt, etc.)	Processed or refined grains (e.g., white rice)	
	Coffee, tea, soda, energy drinks	
	Alcohol	

EXCEPTIONS TO THE RULES

Although we have laid the foundation of what the Bible reveals to us about the Daniel Fast, understand that some individuals may need to make exceptions. If you're pregnant, breastfeeding, or have certain medical needs, seek wisdom in making the right choice for yourself. Ask for wisdom from those around you, and above all, prayerfully follow the Lord's counsel in making decisions that are right for your needs. Don't get caught up in the rules. Get caught up in the opportunity to pursue the Creator of the universe, who will not only supply you with everything you need but also draw closer to you as you press into Him.

Please understand that if you have dietary needs or aren't sure if you can commit to an entire fast, you can still participate! Sacrifice something else you enjoy or simply create a time frame that isn't as overwhelming for you. There is nowhere in scripture that demands you do this a certain way or in a certain time frame. Your desire to grow in a relationship and humble yourself before the Lord is where it all begins.

Water, Not Wine

Water is essential to your health, but water represents more than just physical need. Just as we desire our thirst to be quenched on a daily basis, there is also an innate thirst for something more. Throughout the Bible, water symbolizes many things. Baptism, for example, represents the reborn self being cleansed and raised to a life of walking in faith. In John 4, we are reminded of the Samaritan woman at the well. In Jesus's time, the Jews and Samaritans didn't associate with one another, so when Jesus asked the woman for a drink, she wondered why. Christ presented the Gospel to her like this: "Everyone who drinks this water will be thirsty again, but whoever drinks the water I give them will never thirst. Indeed, the water I give them will become in them a spring of water welling up to eternal life" (John 4:13–14). Drinking solely water during the Daniel Fast is a reminder that although our thirst may never be fully quenched on this earth, we have an eternal spring of water that will never run dry.

WHY DO THE DANIEL FAST?

When I think of fasting, my instinct is to think about hunger. Why would I voluntarily abstain from satisfaction when everything I need is so easily accessible? In his book *Spiritual Disciplines for the Christian Life*, Donald Whitney defines fasting as "a Christian's voluntary abstinence from food for spiritual purposes." Throughout the Bible, there are several instances recorded of people fasting and praying. Why? These people wanted to experience God.

The Daniel Fast is an opportunity to experience God like you never have before. Daniel didn't fast because he wanted people to see him suffering and have pity on him. His goal wasn't to trim down his waistline. Certainly Daniel didn't fast to honor King Nebuchadnezzar. Daniel fasted because he knew that the God he worshipped was his sustainer, his refuge, and his satisfaction.

"Oh, taste and see that the Lord is good!" says Psalm 34:8 (ESV). Would it make sense to argue that Daniel didn't taste or see the goodness of the Lord just because he didn't eat the king's food? We would be foolish to argue this! Daniel experienced much more than the temporary pleasure of fine food. He tasted the holiness, power, and majesty of God, which negated the physical hunger he experienced.

Fasting allowed Daniel to experience the Lord like he never had before, which should be our desire with this fast. We want our spiritual eyes opened to what we have been given for our greatest need, in addition to taking a new step in obedience to Christ. Scripture says, "Come near to God and he will come near to you" (James 4:8). Know that love generates awe-inspiring worship that radically transforms your relationship with the Creator of the universe.

The Daniel Fast and Weight Loss

You might be waiting for me to mention the elephant in the room: Can you lose weight while participating in the Daniel Fast? Quick answer: Yes. But can any quick answer be that easy? You have to check your motivation. Weight loss is definitely one benefit of a plant-based diet. There are other health benefits, too, which I'll discuss later, and those are all positive side effects. However, you must not lose sight of the reason we sought this journey: the pursuit of Christ.

CHOOSE YOUR DANIEL FAST

Following scripture, I've designed two different fast options for you: a 10-day version (like the one in Daniel 1) and a 21-day version (like the one in Daniel 10). In chapters 3 and 4, you'll find a detailed day-by-day meal plan and a devotional for each version.

As you choose your Daniel Fast, ask yourself a couple of questions (and don't feel bad—God wants you to be honest with Him and with yourself). Can I commit to a 10-day or a 21-day fast? Can I drink only water and eat a plant-based diet for the duration? When making this decision, pray to God. If you're committed but you know you, say, can't give up coffee, that's okay. God doesn't want you to fail. Just write it down in your journal.

The Simple 10-Day Daniel Fast

Based on Daniel's first, shorter fast, this version of the Daniel Fast is only 10 days long, and it's all about keeping things simple. This is a perfect choice if you're fasting for the first time or if you don't have a lot of time for food preparation. The 10-day meal plan uses similar ingredients throughout, so you don't have to shop for a bunch of different ingredients or spend too much time in the kitchen. I want to be mindful of your time and your finances. I don't want you to go buy all kinds of grains and end up using only half of each package. The Daniel Fast is about prayer to God—not being stressed about preparing food!

If this is your first Daniel Fast, I'd recommend starting with the 10-day plan. Remember, this is all about your relationship with God, who is "merciful and gracious, slow to anger and abounding in steadfast love" (Psalm 103:8). He loves you and wants you to succeed.

The Flexible 21-Day Daniel Fast

Based on Daniel's second, longer fast, this version of the Daniel Fast is three weeks long and focuses more on flexibility. This plan is a little more creative and varied than the 10-day plan—which is good, because it's three weeks long, so you want to keep it from getting too monotonous. I recommend this version if you have more time for meal preparation or if you've done the Daniel Fast before and feel comfortable committing to 21 days of this way of eating.

Freestyle Daniel Fast

Of course, maybe you don't want to use either of these meal plans! Maybe you're doing this fast with your church or Bible study group and you've agreed on different parameters, or maybe you just have other ideas. That's okay! You can still pick and choose from the recipes in this book, which are all plant-based and suitable for your Daniel Fast.

My prayer for you is to do this fast for however many days you can commit to, so you don't fail and then feel bad about it. You can start with a two-day or five-day fast. Remember, it's more about prayers to Jesus than what you're eating.

If You Stumble

Throughout this journey, I want you to remember why you chose this experience. In the midst of temptation, remember the Lord as your sustainer, the One "who is able to keep you from stumbling and to present you before his glorious presence without fault and with great joy" (Jude 1:24). However, when moments of weakness come, know that it's okay. If you give in to temptation or find yourself in a situation with no options suitable for the Daniel Fast, the Lord knows your heart and desire to pursue Him. Be reminded of His patient love and grace. Seek Him in prayer. If you need to repent, humble yourself before the throne and allow His strength to empower you to start again.

NOURISHING YOUR BODY

"Plant-based diet." Those words can be scary to any meat lover. Can a diet with no animal products really give us everything our body needs? The answer is yes! God has provided us with everything we need through His creation. In fact, if you look at the book of Genesis, plants were the only resource for food in the Garden of Eden: "Then God said, 'I give you every seed-bearing plant on the face of the whole earth and every tree that has fruit with seed in it. They will be yours for food'" (Genesis 1:29).

Studies in peer-reviewed scientific journals like *The American Journal of Clinical Nutrition*, *Nutrients*, and Kaiser Permanente's *The Permanente Journal* have shown that a quality plant-based diet is nutritionally adequate if done correctly. In fact, the health benefits are impressive, as this lifestyle has been linked to a lower risk of conditions like heart disease, diabetes, cancer, obesity, and more. Most plant foods contain proteins; some, like tofu, contain just as much as meat. Long-term vegans often take B_{12} supplements, as it's harder to find in plant-based foods, but this is less of a concern if you're only doing the Daniel Fast for 10 or 21 days.

Nutrition on the Daniel Fast

NUTRIENT	FOOD
VITAMIN A	Carrots, sweet potatoes, spinach, cantaloupes, bell peppers, mangos
VITAMIN C	Bell peppers, broccoli, citrus fruits, strawberries, kiwis, Brussels sprouts
VITAMIN D	Mushrooms, sun exposure
VITAMIN E	Nuts, seeds, tomatoes, spinach, broccoli
CALCIUM	Greens (e.g., spinach, collard, kale, turnip), legumes
FOLATE	Rice, beans, greens, asparagus, Brussels sprouts, avocados, broccoli
PROTEIN	Soy, legumes, nuts, seeds, quinoa, beans, rice
IRON	Legumes, spinach, beet greens
ZINC	Soy, legumes, whole grains, pumpkin seeds, cashews

NOURISHING YOUR SOUL

The Bible calls us to take care of our bodies, because "your body is a temple of the Holy Spirit within you" (1 Corinthians 6:19, ESV). But the Bible also says that "while bodily training is of some value, godliness is of value in every way, as it holds promise for the present life and also for the life to come" (1 Timothy 4:8, ESV).

That is why we are here. We are here to pursue godliness. We are here to pursue a deeper relationship with our Heavenly Father. We are here to come with confidence before the throne of heaven, knowing that the Lord is the satisfying element we need each moment. Jesus said, "Man shall not live by bread alone, but by every word that comes from the mouth of God" (Matthew 4:4). Fasting is meant to draw us closer to Christ.

Think of it this way. To be successful on the Daniel Fast, it's common sense to fill your refrigerator with the types of food you've committed to eating during the fast, right? Filling your kitchen with wine, cheese, and cookies would only position you for failure. The same is true with our spiritual lives. What are we filling our minds with? Are we telling ourselves that the power is within ourselves, or are we trusting that the Lord is our sustainer in the midst of temptation and seeking truth in His word?

As Lysa TerKeurst puts it in her book *Trustworthy: Overcoming Our Greatest Struggles to Trust God*, "Our souls crave to be filled just like our stomachs do. . . . Our souls were made to be nourished by God's Word." If we fed our bodies only every few days, the resulting malnourishment would affect our daily lives. Just as our physical bodies need food to sustain us, our spiritual bodies need the Word of God to sustain us and provide us with what we need to face whatever life throws our way.

Because of this longing, we must set aside time to spend with the Lord. That's why each day of both meal plans in this book includes a short devotion. Take a moment to meditate over these passages, spend time in prayer, and know that His Word will never be void or empty. As you seek to press into the Savior throughout this journey, you will find the satisfaction that your soul has been craving all along.

THE DANIEL FAST IN A GROUP

Proverbs 27:17 says, "Iron sharpens iron, and one man sharpens another" (ESV). Woven throughout scripture are examples of people living life together. Even Christ surrounded Himself with a group of friends. Throughout this time of fasting, surround yourself with people who can hold you accountable and fight the inevitable moments of temptation. There is strength in numbers. Find someone who's willing to push you and who you're willing to encourage throughout this time of commitment. Ask each other how you're doing, where you've struggled, and how you can love, encourage, and lift each other in prayer each day. Walking with someone next to you gives you a strength that you aren't able to experience walking alone.

Remember, it's more about prayers to Jesus than about what you're eating. Do this fast with a friend or your sisterhood or brotherhood group for support. Create a Facebook group to encourage one another and share devotions. Exchange your favorite recipes. "And though a man might prevail against one who is alone, two will withstand him—a threefold cord is not quickly broken" (Ecclesiastes 4:12, ESV).

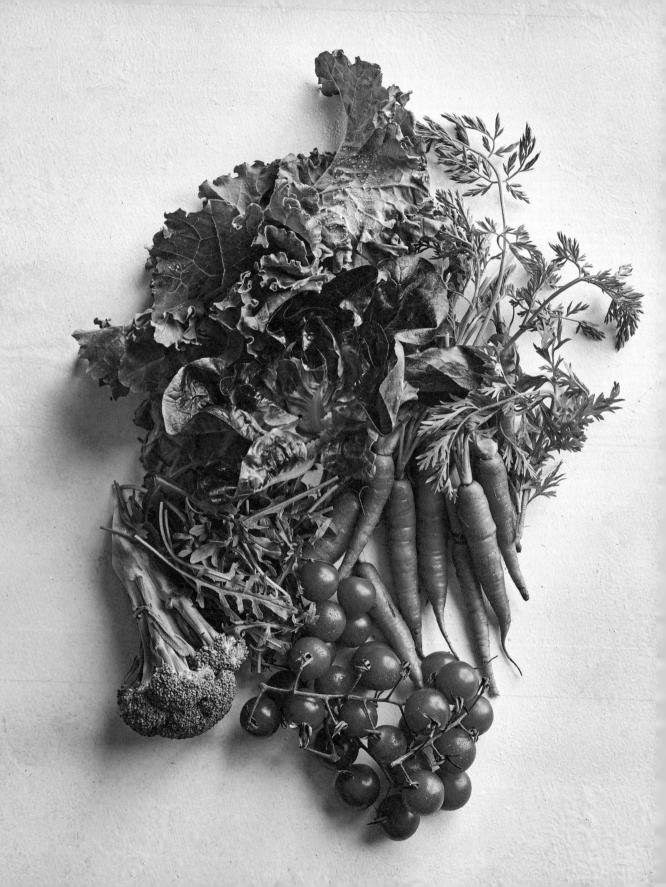

CHAPTER 2

Preparing for the Daniel Fast

Setting yourself up for success is vital to completing the Daniel Fast. Think of it like running a marathon: Without preparation, it would be a miserable endeavor, but with preparation, it can be one of the most rewarding experiences of your life. This chapter will help you navigate the busyness of life in order to prepare yourself for an uninterrupted encounter with your Creator, so you can fully experience what the Lord has in store for you during the Daniel Fast.

STOCKING YOUR PANTRY

Take a look at the 10-day meal plan or the 21-day meal plan. Then make your grocery list based on the recipes you'll be preparing. It may be easier to pick one or two days a week and use them to prepare your food for the rest of the week. You can, for example, cook a lot of quinoa all at once if you know you'll be using it in several recipes in the next few days. Just divide it up into sealable containers and store it in the refrigerator. Another example: roast a bunch of vegetables in advance. They'll stay fresh in the refrigerator for a week in a sealable container. Also be mindful of the costs of grains and vegetables during your fast. Be sure to look at your grocery store's weekly advertisements and check out your local farmers' markets.

KITCHEN EQUIPMENT

These are the kitchen tools you'll find handy, based on the foods you'll be eating and the recipes I'm sharing.

Need-to-Have Items

You probably have many of these kitchen items already. If they've been in the back of your cupboard for a while, take them out and clean them!

Pots and pans. I love my cast-iron pan for cooking vegetables, but any sauté pan will work great.

Baking sheets. You'll be roasting a lot of vegetables! Keep parchment paper on hand for extra-easy clean up.

Cutting board. I suggest using a wooden or bamboo cutting board.

Knives. Remember, sharp knives are safer than dull ones! Invest in a good chef's knife and a paring knife. You'll keep using them long after you complete the Daniel Fast.

Vegetable peeler. This is an inexpensive but necessary tool for peeling your vegetables without any waste—and if you don't have a spiralizer, you'll need a vegetable peeler to turn zucchini into zucchini noodles.

Blender. It doesn't have to be a fancy one! Blenders are great for preparing soups and fresh salad dressings.

Nice-to-Have Items

These items will make your Daniel Fast easier, but if you don't have them, you don't need to go out and buy them all. (Remember, Daniel didn't have any of these modern tools. He didn't even have Trader Joe's!)

Grill basket. You can grill almost any vegetable, and a grill basket lets you do it in bulk. Grill up a bunch of vegetables and enjoy during the week in your salads or lunch bowls.

Food processor. Not all food processors are expensive, and they have so many uses! If you purchase one, choose one that comes with different disks and attachments to chop, shred, mix, and more.

Spiralizer. This handy gadget turns zucchini (and many other vegetables) into spiralized "noodles," which are the same shape and size as spaghetti, but much healthier!

Electric pressure cooker (such as an Instant Pot). This appliance is perfect for a big pot of vegetarian sloppy joes, chili, risotto, or other one-pot recipes. The electric version works fast, and it's much safer than a traditional pressure cooker.

Slow cooker. If you don't have an Instant Pot, a slow cooker does the same work. It just takes longer. Just get it started before you leave the house, and dinner will be ready when you get home!

How to Cook Vegetables

METHOD	PURPOSE	WHICH VEGGIES WORK BEST
ROASTING	Roasting vegetables at 400–425°F is the easiest and most flavorful way to cook them. Roasting gives vegetables a crispy texture as their natural flavors develop. For maximum convenience, prepare all your vegetables in advance, and then roast them all at once. A baking sheet(s) and parchment paper is all you need!	Acorn squash, asparagus, beets, bell pepper, broccoli, Brussels sprouts, butternut squash, cabbage, carrots, cauliflower, eggplant, fennel, green beans, kale, mushrooms, onions, parsnips, potatoes, squash, sweet potatoes, tomatoes, turnips, zucchini.
STEAMING	Steaming is the healthiest method to cook your vegetables because it doesn't use any fat. Steamed vegetables are great for a side dish, bowl, or salad. You can simply squeeze fresh lemon over the vegetables to add extra flavor.	You can steam most vegetables, except a few like tomatoes, bell peppers, eggplant, and mushrooms.
SAUTÉING	Sautéing means cooking food in a pan with a small amount of fat (like olive oil or coconut oil) over medium-high heat. Sautéing is a quicker way to cook, but it requires more attention than roasting or steaming.	Pretty much all vegetables.

GOING WITHOUT

Recently, a friend told me, "I'm fearful of God taking away what I love." Although we may not voice this, I believe many of us hold on to things because we fear what would happen if they were no longer a part of our lives. We've convinced ourselves that this desire is a *need*, created in order to fill something in us that is lacking. However, the truth is that only Christ can fill those voids.

Daniel provides an example of going without in order that the Lord would fulfill in Daniel what only He could do. In these moments of sacrifice and submission, Daniel encountered the Lord. With each fast, the Lord provided abundantly for Daniel. And that same God who was with Daniel is with you also. If you do give in to temptation, use these moments to press into the Lord, asking Him to satisfy those cravings and fill in you what only He can fill.

Let's take a look at several food items most people find difficult to give up, remembering that our ultimate goal is more of Christ Himself and trusting in the Lord to quench the desires that have the potential to hinder our experience with Him.

No Meat

Although giving up meat can be a challenge, there are many alternatives to satisfy our hunger and provide us with the nutrients we need. Temptations will come, so in those moments, remember the Lord's faithfulness to Daniel, knowing that He will give you everything you need. After Daniel and his friends ate only vegetables and water for 10 days, they were not only physically healthier—they also gained knowledge and skills (Daniel 1:17).

No Dairy or Eggs

In addition to foods like scrambled eggs or cheese and crackers, many of us enjoy milk with our cereal or creamer in our coffee. These smaller luxuries may tempt you to break your fast, but remember, in the midst of temptation, the Lord can satisfy your longing: "The Lord is my shepherd, I shall not want" (Psalm 23:1, KJV). There are also many alternative options for dairy and egg products. Though the recipes in this book don't use the processed, factory-made vegan products available in stores, the recipes will tell you how to make your own nut milks and flax eggs. Soaking cashews in water for a few hours gives them a nice creamy texture when blended into sauces or soups.

No Sugar

While in ancient times sugar was regarded as a luxury, it has thoroughly permeated modern food. If you have a sweet tooth, keeping a bowl of fresh fruit can help satisfy that craving for something sweet and help you endure the temptations that will come your way. Don't allow the desires of this world to overwhelm your longing to draw closer to Christ. The apostle Paul was content in Christ even when he was imprisoned for his faith (which was probably harder than going without sugar for a few weeks!). "I have learned to be content whatever the circumstances," he wrote. "I know what it is to be in need, and I know what it is to have plenty. I have learned the secret of being content in any and every situation, whether well fed or hungry, whether living in plenty or in want. I can do all this through him who gives me strength" (Philippians 4:11–13).

No Caffeine

Most of us have a source of caffeine we gravitate toward. From soda to coffee to energy drinks, we find ourselves trying to beat any crashes in energy we might feel throughout the day. Our reliance on these drinks is high, making this sacrifice seem almost impossible for some. When you find yourself tempted, know that your relationship with the Lord is far more desirable than a temporary fill, because "everyone who drinks of this water will be thirsty again, but whoever drinks of the water that I will give him will never be thirsty again" (John 4:13–14, ESV). And remember: If you need to set the rules of your Daniel Fast to allow decaf coffee and herbal tea in addition to water, that's better than failing at the Daniel Fast and becoming discouraged.

Snacking on the Daniel Fast

Although you should be a little hungry during the Daniel Fast, snacking is allowed. It just shouldn't consist of "choice foods" or "delicacies," like potato chips or sugary granola bars. See chapter 9 for fast-compliant snacks and side dishes, or keep vegetables and fruits ready to go for those "too hungry to function" moments. Some simple ideas include apple slices with all-natural peanut butter or carrot sticks with homemade hummus.

WHEN YOU CAN'T COOK

Working overtime, late-in-the-day soccer practice, scheduled outings—many life circumstances can make it difficult to find time to cook a meal. But don't worry. You can still stick to the Daniel Fast.

Ordering at a Restaurant

Depending on your social life, it may be unrealistic to avoid restaurants completely, especially if you're doing the 21-day fast. If you're going to a restaurant, try to be prepared, remember your limitations, and honor the commitment you've made during these days. Many restaurants have their menus posted online, so go ahead and scan the menu ahead of time. If none of the entrees fit the fast, look for a salad or side dish that does. Just make sure that the salad dressing is vegan. If you have questions, ask them. I know from experience that this can save you from eating something outside of the fasting recommendations.

Packaged Food

Although you have to be careful, some packaged foods are available on the Daniel Fast. Frozen vegetables, unsalted nuts, and any dried fruits with no added sugars or preservatives can be eaten on this diet. But watch out. If you read the labels, many seemingly natural or plant-based products contain ingredients that aren't Daniel Fast–friendly. Make yourself aware of your purchases, and you'll quickly learn how to maintain this fast without your normal choices.

Other Ways to Take a Break from Cooking

All of us get tired of making meals daily, but because the Daniel Fast only happens for a limited amount of time, it's easier to prepare foods ahead of time for those days when cooking isn't possible.

- Double a recipe and put the leftovers in the fridge for tomorrow—or in the freezer for a ready-to-heat meal later on.

- If you're doing the Daniel Fast in a group, get together and prepare meals with one another to get ready for your journey.

- Organize a potluck at your church or within your group for which everybody brings a little something.

Tips, Tricks, and Reminders

Here are some tips and tricks to help you achieve the best results during your Daniel Fast.

- Do the Daniel Fast for the number of days that you can commit to, so you don't fail and become discouraged. If this is your first Daniel Fast, go with the 10-day version. You can even start with a two-day or five-day fast.
- Look at the meal plans in chapters 3 and 4 (or write your own meal plan), and make a grocery list. Buy grains and nonperishables in bulk, but get your vegetables fresh every week. (Frozen vegetables work, too!)
- Pick one day each week to do meal preparation ahead of time. You can make extra rice or extra roasted veggies on that day to use in new recipes on those days when you have less time.
- Be sure to drink plenty of water!
- Keep a bowl of fresh fruit available to grab from during the day.

SOME LAST WORDS OF ENCOURAGEMENT

The Daniel Fast always brings me to a whole new spiritual level. My physical and emotional health also increase. It won't always be easy, but you've got this. The first few days are the hardest. Keep praying! You're doing this for a greater reason: to deepen your relationship with God through reliance on Him.

Put up a prayer board and use it each day. Keep a journal with you at all times, and use it to write down your prayers, thoughts, and what you eat each day. Share this journey with a friend or a family member. If you're fasting with a group, plan on connecting every couple of days to encourage one another, pray together, and, of course, sit down to eat together! I lean on my sisterhood group for any ups and downs. I am excited for what God has in store for you. Stay committed and faith will find you!

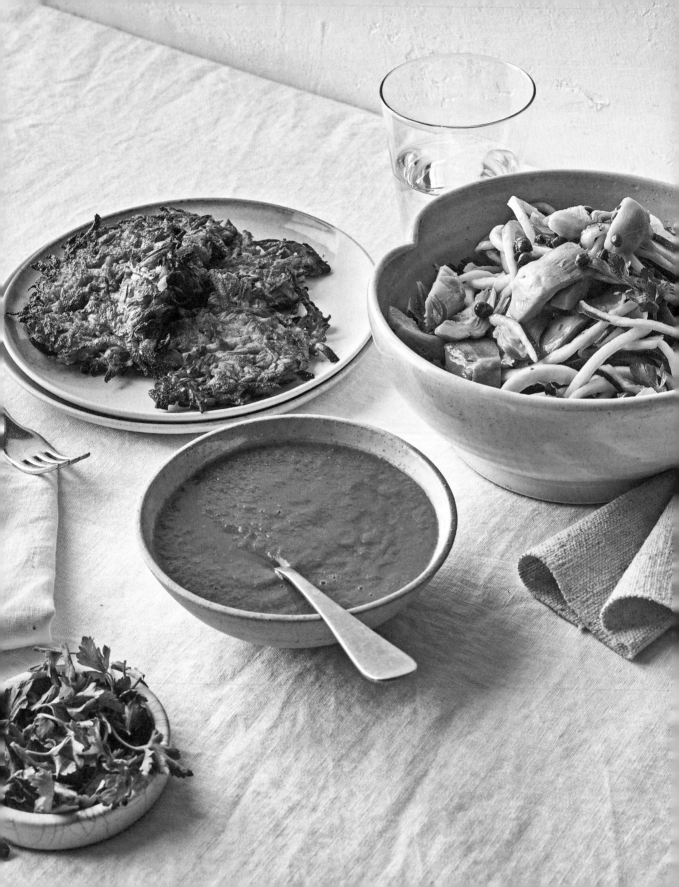

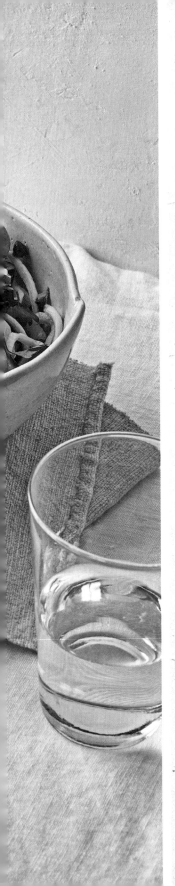

PART II

DANIEL FAST MEAL PLANS

AND

DEVOTIONALS

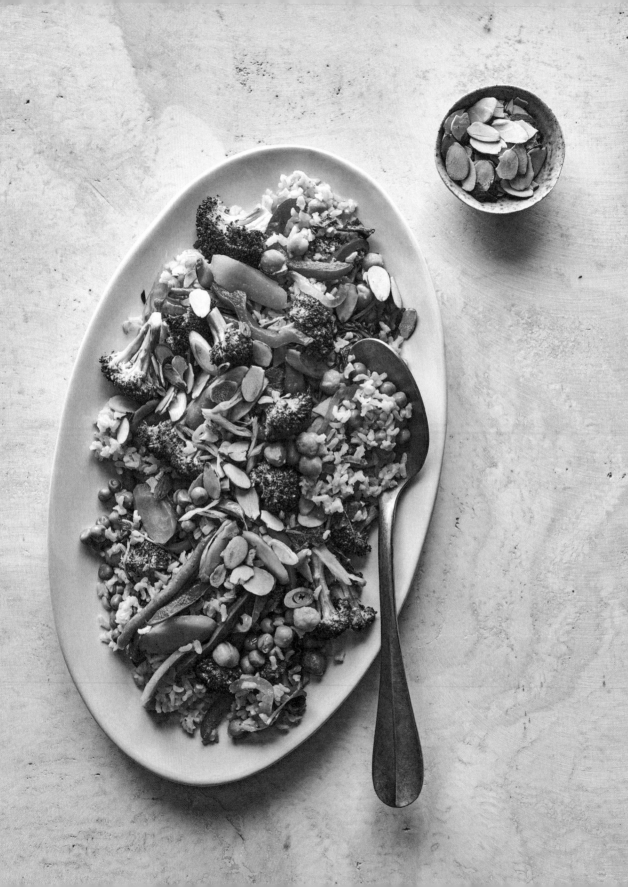

CHAPTER 3

The Simple 10-DAY Daniel Fast Meal Plan and Devotional

This 10-day Daniel Fast, based on the one described in Daniel 1, is perfect for people who are newer to the Daniel Fast. Not only is this plan shorter, it also focuses on simpler recipes, so that you can devote more mental energy to God and less to food. This chapter has a meal plan and a devotion for all 10 days. Eat, pray, and enjoy!

‹ Ginger-Sesame Vegetable Stir-Fry, page 110

DAY 1

But when you fast, put oil on your head and wash your face, so that it will not be obvious to others that you are fasting, but only to your Father, who is unseen; and your Father, who sees what is done in secret, will reward you.

MATTHEW 6:17-18

It's easy to look at fasting and see what we're lacking rather than what we're gaining. However, our fasting has a purpose, and we must be willing to check our mindset daily. Overwhelming our desire for radical transformation by idolizing a need for cultural approval hinders our ability to experience what we're longing for. Without pursuing Christ in this process, we will find ourselves going hungry with no spiritual gain. Trust that He is working in the inner parts of your heart to draw you closer to Himself today.

BREAKFAST:
Customizable Overnight Oats (page 68)

LUNCH:
Lentil Greek Salad (page 89)

MIDDAY SNACK:
Handful of unsalted almonds

DINNER:
Quinoa and Black Bean Burger (page 111) with Italian Chopped Salad (page 87)

DAY 2

So after they had fasted and prayed, they placed their hands on them and sent them off.

ACTS 13:3

Daniel chose to abstain from ordinary foods because he had experienced the power of the Lord. Just think of this: At this point in his life, the Lord had delivered him and his friends from the king's lordship over them. They had been delivered from the fiery furnace. And the mouths of a den of lions had been closed because Daniel knew that his God was able to do immeasurably more than he could imagine. Everything culture told Daniel he needed was nothing in comparison with what he knew he already had. Fasting brings us to a place of longing for and remembering the faithfulness of the God we serve. Allow this to draw you closer to Him today.

BREAKFAST:
Chickpea-Flax "Omelet"
with Spinach and Scallions
(page 72)

LUNCH:
Make-Ahead Quinoa Salad
in a Jar (page 90)

MIDDAY SNACK:
Banana and a scoop
of all-natural nut butter

DINNER:
Eggplant-Wrapped Veggie
"Meat Loaf" (page 112)
with Sweet Potato Latkes
(page 139)

DAY 3

There was also a prophet, Anna.... She never left the temple but worshiped night and day, fasting and praying.

LUKE 2:36–37

All of us are seeking something to fill the places in our hearts that feel empty. However, if we look to the things of this world, we will constantly find ourselves aching, wondering why we aren't satisfied. In her book *Uninvited*, Lysa TerKeurst writes that God "waits every day with every answer we need, every comfort we crave, every affection we're desperate for, while we look everywhere else but at Him.... How it must break His heart ... *the world entices our flesh but never embraces our soul*" (emphasis mine). Those things we crave? The Lord is longing to fill them. But without Him, we'll never understand the true embrace of the One who is everything we need. Look to Him today. Rest in Him, seek Him, be still with Him, and allow Him to saturate your soul with His presence today.

BREAKFAST:
Customizable Overnight Oats
(page 68)

LUNCH:
Brown Rice, Mushroom, and
Kale Soup (page 81)

MIDDAY SNACK:
Chopped carrots and celery
(dipped in all-natural
nut butter)

DINNER:
Italian Lentil "Meatballs"
(page 114) over
zucchini noodles

DAY 4

Yet when they were ill, I put on sackcloth and humbled myself with fasting. When my prayers returned to me unanswered, I went about mourning as though for my friend or brother. I bowed my head in grief as though weeping for my mother.

PSALM 35:13–14

Fasting creates an earnestness in prayer that is difficult to emulate through any other experience. It exposes our need for the satisfying Savior and the stage of our helplessness without Him. In an interview on his website, DesiringGod.org, pastor and author John Piper said, "Fasting is a physical exclamation point at the end of our pleas to God. It says, 'I need you! I want you! You are my treasure!' . . . We fast to express our longing or our ache for all the implications of Jesus's power in the present moment that isn't completely realized." Seek His power to work radically in your life today and know that He is the only one who can fill the longing of your soul.

BREAKFAST:
Blueberry-Lemon Oatmeal
Muffins (page 70)

LUNCH:
Italian Chopped Salad
(page 87)

MIDDAY SNACK:
Fresh fruit

DINNER:
Fiesta Rice Bowl with Tofu
(page 96)

DAY 5

This is the confidence we have in approaching God: that if we ask anything according to his will, he hears us.

1 JOHN 5:14

In the same interview about fasting quoted in yesterday's devotion, John Piper says, "We want to see people healed. We want to see people saved. We want to see marriages redeemed. We ache, and we long for this to happen; therefore, we ask Jesus to come by putting this exclamation point of longing at the end of our desires." The Lord knows the desires of our hearts. How humbling is it that the Creator of the universe cares for us enough to listen to our requests? Approach His throne today with humility, confidence, and expectancy, knowing that He hears you and will answer according to His will and timing.

BREAKFAST:
Granola Bites (page 69)

LUNCH:
Lentil Greek Salad (page 89)

MIDDAY SNACK:
White Bean Hummus
(page 141) with
sliced vegetables

DINNER:
Lentil Shepherd's Pie
(page 126)

DAY 6

But when you pray, go into your room, close the door and pray to your Father, who is unseen. Then your Father, who sees what is done in secret, will reward you. And when you pray, do not keep on babbling like pagans, for they think they will be heard because of their many words. Do not be like them, for your Father knows what you need before you ask him.

MATTHEW 6:6–8

Isn't it amazing to know that even before we ask, the Father knows what we need? Some wonder, "If that's true, why even bother asking?" However, prayer is vital to the life of every Christian. Not only does it deepen our relationship with the Lord, it also allows us to experience everything He has to offer. Through prayer, He reveals Himself to us on a personal level. Some of my most precious moments with my Creator have been those tucked away in the quietness of my apartment. Overwhelmed with His presence, the longing in my heart is satisfied. And looking back at His faithfulness throughout my life helps me to know that He is working, even in the places I cannot see. Walk in confidence today, knowing that He will supply everything you need for each moment as you submit your life to Him.

BREAKFAST:
Tofu Scramble Breakfast Bowl
(page 74)

LUNCH:
Leftover Lentil Shepherd's Pie
(page 126)

MIDDAY SNACK:
White Bean Hummus
(page 141) with sliced celery
and carrots

DINNER:
Italian Lentil "Meatballs"
(page 114) with Italian
Chopped Salad (page 87)

DAY 7

Ask and it will be given to you; seek and you will find.... Which of you fathers, if your son asks for a fish, will give him a snake instead? Or if he asks for an egg, will give him a scorpion? If you then, though you are evil, know how to give good gifts to your children, how much more will your Father in heaven give the Holy Spirit to those who ask him!

LUKE 11:9–13

Being a parent was the hardest job life could ever bring me, but also the most rewarding. As a single mother, it wasn't always easy. When my son asked for the sneakers all the other kids had, I did my best to make sure he got them. My daughter was in cheerleading and it was extremely expensive. Therefore I worked two jobs. This scripture really brings life as a parent home for me. I couldn't imagine giving my children anything but what they love. This is what the Father does for us. When we come to Him in prayer, seek His desires, and walk in obedience, He will open the door and show us the good gifts He has for us. Pursue Him today, and run with open arms to the One who will always give you what you need.

BREAKFAST:
Customizable Overnight Oats
(page 68)

LUNCH:
Leftover Italian Lentil
"Meatballs" (page 114)
with vegetables

MIDDAY SNACK:
Handful of nuts

DINNER:
Ginger-Sesame Vegetable
Stir-Fry (page 110)

DAY 8

If any of you lacks wisdom, you should ask God, who gives generously to all without finding fault, and it will be given to you.

JAMES 1:5

Wisdom is mentioned throughout scripture. In 2 Chronicles, Solomon prays for wisdom after taking his father's throne. Ecclesiastes 9:18 says that "wisdom is better than weapons of war," and James 3:17 describes wisdom as "first of all pure; then peace-loving, considerate, submissive, full of mercy and good fruit, impartial and sincere."

But how do we get this wisdom? All we have to do is ask! How amazing is it that this supernatural gift is available to us if we simply ask for it? Can you imagine being Daniel and having ten times more wisdom than anyone in the kingdom? Me neither! But the God who was with Daniel throughout his time under the king is the very same God we have access to this very day. Take time to seek His wisdom and understanding as you pursue His Kingdom today.

BREAKFAST:
Lemon Energy Pancakes
(page 76)

LUNCH:
Green Goodness Superfood
Bowl with Avocado (page 101)

MIDDAY SNACK:
Zucchini Chips (page 137)

DINNER:
Peanut-Lime Rice Bowl
(page 105)

DAY 9

When they had assembled at Mizpah, they drew water and poured it out before the Lord. On that day they fasted and there they confessed, "We have sinned against the Lord."

1 SAMUEL 7:6

Although it is sometimes difficult to see the Old Testament as scripture we can identify with, I believe it's much more relatable than we often think. The Israelites had a history of idol worship, valuing tangible "gods" over the true Creator. There is a common consensus among many theological leaders today that we become what we worship, and this worship can lead to ruin or restoration. As you continue to follow this journey, are there areas in your life where you're placing something else before the King of Kings? Are you worshiping the created rather than the Creator? Come to the Lord in prayer and allow Him to move in you, entrusting Him to open your heart to pursue Him over anything else.

BREAKFAST:
Sweet Potato Breakfast Muffins (page 75)

LUNCH:
Vegan Faux Pho (page 84)

MIDDAY SNACK:
Buffalo Cauliflower Dip (page 143) with vegetables

DINNER:
Vegetable-Hummus Collard Wrap (page 125) with Sweet Potato Latkes (page 139)

DAY 10

With God all things are possible.

MATTHEW 19:26

So many times, we allow our circumstances to overshadow what we know the Lord can do. The Bible reminds us that the Lord's thoughts and ways are higher than ours (Isaiah 55:8) and that "no purpose of [His] can be thwarted" (Job 42:2). Don't allow fear to keep you from taking a step in faith. Because with you in that step is a God who will be everything you need—the net you land in, the wings you soar on, the strength you need—no matter what happens.

I want to congratulate you on walking through this 10-day journey! I'm sure there were moments where you weren't sure if you would make it, but here you are on the other side. Take some time to reflect on the Lord's sustaining grace over the last week and a half. Allow it to bring you to a place of humility and awe-inspired worship that He is who He says He is. Don't allow your pursuit of Him to stop here. This is only a dot in the expanse of what He has for you!

BREAKFAST:
Fruit-Topped Chickpea Crepes
(page 71)

LUNCH:
Quinoa Veggie Bowl
(page 100)

MIDDAY SNACK:
Leftover Sweet Potato Latkes
(page 139)

DINNER:
Fava Bean and Mushroom
"Pot Roast" (page 130)

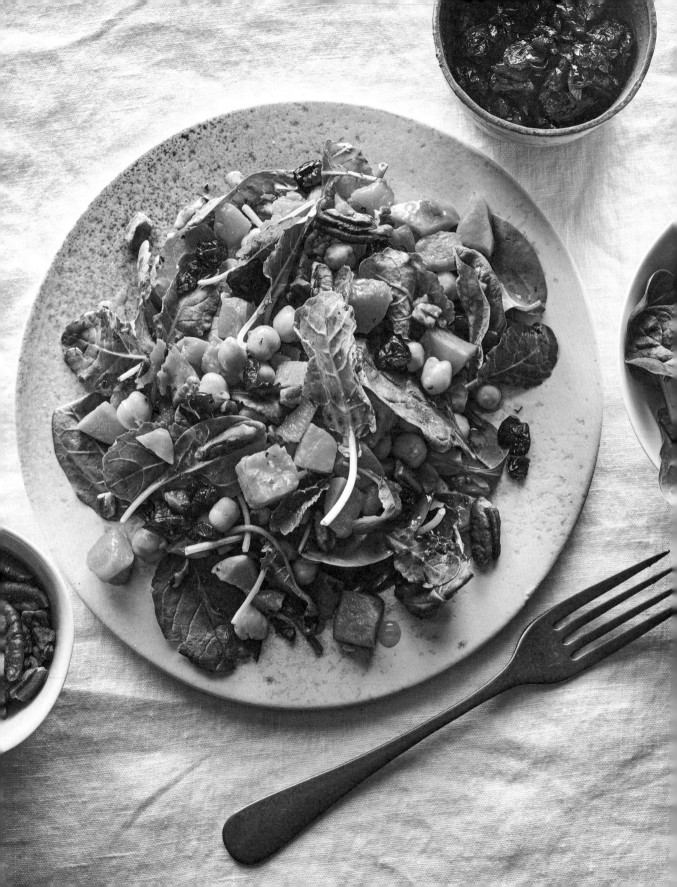

CHAPTER 4

The Flexible 21-DAY Daniel Fast Meal Plan and Devotional

This 21-day Daniel Fast is based on the one described in Daniel 10. While it's a bit more challenging than the 10-day Daniel Fast, it also offers more variety and creativity in what you'll be eating. It's a great fit if you have some experience with the Daniel Fast or if you have more time for meal preparation and cooking. This chapter contains a meal plan and devotion for all 21 days. I pray that the Lord will soften your heart and give you the strength to endure through this journey.

< Power Greens with Roasted Butternut Squash, page 88

DAY 1

He must become greater; I must become less.

JOHN 3:30

Although this is my favorite verse in the Bible, many days I am challenged with whether I am truly living it or not. Many religious practices call us to self-edification or self-improvement, but this verse calls us to just the opposite. Looking at the life of Christ, we see a servant heart, a humble spirit, and a desire to love even the people society considered the lowliest.

Philippians 2:7 even says that He "made himself nothing by taking the very nature of a servant, being made in human likeness." Through His testimony, we are called to be His ambassadors, seeking to live our lives as He did. Today, I want to challenge you to evaluate those things in your life that tend to become greater than God. Ask Him to loosen the fists you're holding so tightly and allow Him to open your hands in submission to Him.

BREAKFAST:
Chickpea-Flax "Omelet"
with Spinach and Scallions
(page 72)

LUNCH:
Italian Chopped Salad
(page 87)

MIDDAY SNACK:
Handful of unsalted almonds

DINNER:
Mediterranean Casserole
(page 117)

DAY 2

One thing I ask from the Lord, this only do I seek: that I may dwell in the house of the Lord all the days of my life, to gaze on the beauty of the Lord and to see him in his temple.

PSALM 27:4

Walking by myself makes me more aware of my surroundings. It's so beautiful to see God's hand in the creation around me. Sometimes I'm led to stop in my tracks and take in the moment. Has that ever happened to you? When we gaze on something, we look at it intently without taking our eyes off it. We can sometimes lose track of time, as we are mesmerized by the beauty of the scene. I pray that we would not miss the opportunity to fix our gaze on the beauty of today.

There is nothing more lovely than to gaze upon the beauty of Christ. He is the essence of beauty, and to fix our gaze on Him is to remove ourselves from the distractions around us. He is inherently beautiful, and what He has accomplished is immeasurably more mesmerizing than anything that surrounds us. My prayer for you today is that you would know what it means to fix your gaze upon the beauty of the Lord and that He would overwhelm all that you are, filling you with His presence.

BREAKFAST:
Customizable Overnight Oats
(page 68)

LUNCH:
Fiesta Rice Bowl with Tofu
(page 96)

MIDDAY SNACK:
Banana and a scoop of
all-natural nut butter

DINNER:
Mediterranean Vegetables
over Spaghetti Squash
(page 123)

DAY 3

I, Daniel, was the only one who saw the vision; those who were with me did not see it, but such terror overwhelmed them that they fled and hid themselves.

DANIEL 10:7

The God who revealed Himself to Daniel is the same God who hears your requests today. Rather than running in fear as Daniel's companions did, stand in humility before His throne, knowing that Christ is interceding on your behalf. The Lord knows our words before they come out of our mouths, and as we seek His direction, we must take time to be still and listen. Set aside time today to approach the throne with an open and humble heart, asking the Lord to reveal Himself like never before. And when He does, allow His strength to empower you as you press onward to answer His calling.

BREAKFAST:
Blueberry-Lemon Oatmeal Muffins (page 70)

LUNCH:
Power Greens with Roasted Butternut Squash (page 88)

MIDDAY SNACK:
Chopped carrots and celery (dipped in all-natural nut butter)

DINNER:
Very Veggie Layer Lasagna (page 118) and Italian Chopped Salad (page 87)

DAY 4

The wicked flee though no one pursues, but the righteous are as bold as a lion.

PROVERBS 28:1

Measured at 114 decibels, the roar of a lion is pretty intense. (In fact, it's loud enough to cause hearing loss!) God is not calling us to be as *loud* as a lion, but He is calling us to that level of boldness. The Hebrew word for "bold" in this verse is *yivtakh*, and it can also be translated as "confident" or "secure." When we have confidence in something, we are bold. Remember the sure and steadfast anchor you have in Christ today, and pray for the boldness that is yours in Him. Then, seek opportunities to share the gospel story of Christ with others, because it is through His victory on the cross that you carry the hope of eternity.

BREAKFAST:
Lemon Energy Pancakes
(page 76)

LUNCH:
Leftover Very Veggie Layer
Lasagna (page 118)

MIDDAY SNACK:
Leftover Blueberry-Lemon
Oatmeal Muffins (page 70)

DINNER:
Crispy Cauliflower Super Bowl
(page 98) and Zucchini Chips
(page 137)

DAY 5

Shadrach, Meshach, and Abednego answered and said to the king, "O Nebuchadnezzar, we have no need to answer you in this matter. If this be so, our God whom we serve is able to deliver us from the burning fiery furnace, and he will deliver us out of your hand, O king. But if not, be it known to you, O king, that we will not serve your gods or worship the golden image that you have set up."

DANIEL 3:16–18 (ESV)

King Nebuchadnezzar wanted the Jewish people to worship his golden statue. At 90 feet high and 9 feet wide, this idol would be difficult to miss. Those who did give in and worship did so out of a fear of being thrown into the fiery furnace, not because it was their desire. Have you ever felt that way? Have you felt the pressure to do something you didn't want to do? To buy something you didn't have the money for? To eat something because, well, "You only live once!" We become what we worship, and this worship can lead to ruin or restoration. But there were those who didn't give in, and when they were thrown in the fiery furnace, God protected them. Just as Shadrach, Meshach, and Abednego experienced, we have the opportunity to be restored from the fire. Don't allow what you worship to bring you to ruin. Rather, seek the One who is able to make you new.

BREAKFAST:
Customizable Overnight Oats
(page 68)

LUNCH:
Roasted Tomato and Red
Pepper Soup (page 82)

MIDDAY SNACK:
White Bean Hummus
(page 141) with
sliced vegetables

DINNER:
Portabella Mushrooms with
Cashew Ricotta (page 124) and
Roasted Vegetable Medley
(page 138)

DAY 6

Keep your lives free from the love of money and be content with what you have, because God has said, "Never will I leave you; never will I forsake you." So we say with confidence, "The Lord is my helper, I will not be afraid. What can mere mortals do to me?"

HEBREWS 13:5–6

We all want more—more money, a bigger house, a newer car, the most expensive clothes. Our culture promises us that this kind of lifestyle will bring us fulfillment. What we find, however, is that it is a constant pursuit of emptiness. As Christians, our satisfaction lies in the foundational truths of the revealed Word of God. Look at the promise from the Lord in today's verse: "Never will I leave you; never will I forsake you." The fancy house will need repairs, and the fashionable clothes will go out of style. But the God we serve will be with us the same today as He will be 30 or 50 or 100 years from now. Rest in the truth that His presence will never leave you, and seek to find your satisfaction in all that He is.

BREAKFAST:
Sweet Potato and Brussels Sprouts Hash (page 73)

LUNCH:
Italian Farro Bowl (page 95) topped with Pesto with Walnuts (page 149)

MIDDAY SNACK:
White Bean Hummus (page 141) with sliced celery and carrots

DINNER:
Farro and Vegetable Sauté (page 128)

DAY 7

Love is patient, love is kind. It does not envy, it does not boast, it is not proud.

1 CORINTHIANS 13:4

I pray through this verse often. Jesus was crucified for our freedom, which is a display of the true meaning of love. In today's world, we are often jealous of others because they seem to have a better career, to hang out with the popular crowd, or to live an easier life. In a consumer-driven world, it's hard to count our blessings when it feels like we're constantly behind. However, know that just as the Lord has given gifts to the people around you, He has blessed you with His good gifts as well. Stand confident in what He has given you and know that you are divinely placed by Him for this moment. God has a plan for all of us, so rest in His provision over your life.

Today you're one-third of the way through the Daniel Fast! I encourage you to continue writing in your journal and asking the Lord to give you endurance over the next two weeks.

BREAKFAST:
Fruit-Topped Chickpea Crepes
(page 71)

LUNCH:
Power Greens with Roasted
Butternut Squash (page 88)

MIDDAY SNACK:
5-Layer Guacamole Dip
(page 142) with vegetables

DINNER:
Quinoa and Black Bean
Burger (page 111) with
Vegetarian Fried Cauliflower
Rice (page 144)

DAY 8

The Lord does not look at the things people look at. People look at the outward appearance, but the Lord looks at the heart.

1 SAMUEL 16:7

Do you remember the story of King David? David was never believed to be in line for the throne. Overlooked by his own father, David wasn't even brought in from the fields when Samuel was sent to anoint a king from his house. David had no idea that he would go from shepherd to armor-bearer to being persecuted by Saul to becoming king. But God didn't care that David was the youngest of his brothers with the unglamorous job of tending sheep. He cared that David declared his confidence in the One who held his life in His hands. We can't let our circumstances dictate what we can do; only the Lord can do that. So don't be afraid to take steps in faith like the Daniel Fast. God will provide what you need.

BREAKFAST:
Tofu Scramble Breakfast Bowl
(page 74)

LUNCH:
Green Goodness Superfood
Bowl with Avocado (page 101)

MIDDAY SNACK:
Leftover 5-Layer Guacamole
Dip (page 142) with vegetables

DINNER:
Mediterranean Vegetables
over Spaghetti Squash
(page 123)

DAY 9

But we have this treasure in jars of clay to show that this all-surpassing power is from God and not from us.

2 CORINTHIANS 4:7

My one-year-old niece has a plush bunny that she got on the day she was born. This little guy would make even the torn-up Velveteen Rabbit look brand-new. He's her best friend. He's there when she sleeps and there when she wakes up. After a basketball game a few weeks ago, when her family got home, the bunny was nowhere to be found. If you're a parent, you may know how this goes. My niece hardly slept, in tears throughout the night because her friend was gone. The next morning, my sister went back to the gym to look one more time, and the bunny was there! I got a video later that morning of its return, and the way my niece grabbed her friend and smiled would melt anyone's heart. But I got to thinking: Where do my treasures lie? Am I holding on to the treasure of the gospel that has been gifted to me as dearly as my niece held on to that bunny? Today, take an honest look at what you cherish, remembering that we hold the most valuable treasure in the world.

BREAKFAST:
Customizable Overnight Oats (page 68)

LUNCH:
Hearty Tuscan Chili (page 86)

MIDDAY SNACK:
Handful of unsalted almonds

DINNER:
Eggplant-Wrapped Veggie "Meat Loaf" (page 112) with Chilled Tomato and Basil Salad (page 91)

DAY 10

Go, gather together all the Jews who are in Susa, and fast for me. Do not eat or drink for three days, night or day. I and my attendants will fast as you do. When this is done, I will go to the king, even though it is against the law. And if I perish, I perish.

ESTHER 4:16

Through my sisterhood Bible study, I learned about the amazing woman Esther was. In the midst of difficult circumstances, she became queen to King Ahasuerus. Shortly after her reign began, a law was passed that legalized the genocide of the Jewish people. Although she was queen, none of the officials knew she was Jewish, even her husband. This put Esther in a dangerous position. However, Esther believed her God would go before her as she dedicated herself to fasting and prayer. She believed that He could deliver her from the dangers that surrounded her. In the Lord's sovereignty over these difficult circumstances, He provided an opening for Esther to step in and ultimately save her people. Isn't the Lord's power amazing? Take a second today and think about a moment in your life when something you believed was a dead end turned out to be an opening for the Lord to display His miraculous work.

BREAKFAST:
Chickpea-Flax "Omelet" with Spinach and Scallions (page 72)

LUNCH:
Crunchy Nut and Quinoa Bowl (page 102)

MIDDAY SNACK:
Zucchini Chips (page 137)

DINNER:
Fava Bean and Mushroom "Pot Roast" (page 130)

DAY 11

But Ananias answered, "Lord, I have heard from many about this man, how much evil he has done to your saints at Jerusalem." ... But the Lord said to him, "Go, for he is a chosen instrument of mine to carry my name before the Gentiles and kings and the children of Israel."

ACTS 9:13, 15 (ESV)

The apostle Paul started out persecuting Christians. He believed he was doing work that pleased the Lord, so he felt no remorse or guilt. But on his way to Damascus to bind more Christians, he was radically transformed by the Lord and became His chosen instrument to carry the gospel of Jesus Christ to the Gentiles. This conversion reminds us that you don't have to be the "right kind of person" to experience God. If you are sitting in regret, sin, shame, disappointment, or the like, know that the Lord will still draw you to Himself. He's not looking for specific kinds of people. He works through all kinds of situations and people to create a turning point for eternity. Confess your sins, repent, and call on the name of the Lord to rescue your longing heart today. It's never too late to feel the loving embrace of your Heavenly Father.

BREAKFAST:
Sweet Potato and Brussels Sprouts Hash (page 73)

LUNCH:
Roasted Tomato and Red Pepper Soup (page 82)

MIDDAY SNACK:
Roasted Mushrooms (page 136)

DINNER:
Mediterranean Casserole (page 117) with Roasted Acorn Squash with Kale and Pecans (page 140)

DAY 12

All who fear the Lord will hate evil. Therefore, I hate pride and arrogance, corruption and perverse speech.

PROVERBS 8:13 (NLT)

The Biblical concept of "fearing the Lord" is commonly misunderstood. The Hebrew word translated as "fear" here is *yirat*, which can also be translated as "awe." It connotes a humble reverence toward the majesty of God. He is unmatched, and we know His sovereignty is over all things. As we walk in obedience with the Lord, we begin to hate what He hates. We earnestly seek to do what brings Him honor so that His name can be magnified. There are moments where we give in to temptation, but our God provided salvation that exemplifies His perfect, unconditional love. Seek this Truth today, knowing that giving ourselves to Him is a lifelong process of pursuing Him with all we have.

BREAKFAST:
Customizable Overnight Oats
(page 68)

LUNCH:
Leftover Mediterranean
Casserole (page 117) and
Roasted Acorn Squash with
Kale and Pecans (page 140)

MIDDAY SNACK:
Fresh fruit

DINNER:
Mushroom Stroganoff with
Zucchini Ribbons (page 122)

DAY 13

And in every matter of wisdom and understanding about which the king inquired of them, he found them ten times better than all the magicians and enchanters in his whole kingdom.

DANIEL 1:20

Have you ever watched young children put a puzzle together? I'm talking about two- or three-year-olds playing with one of those wooden puzzles where you grab the knob on a puzzle piece and place it where it fits. The children might understand where the piece is supposed to go but be unable to make the edges line up and put it in its place. Frustrated, they come to you with an outstretched hand, asking for help. When the piece is perfectly placed, the biggest smile comes across their faces . . . until they can't figure out the next piece, and the process starts all over again. But in time, they begin to place the pieces by themselves. Eventually, they're able to take what they've learned from that little wooden puzzle and apply it to other puzzles that are more difficult to figure out.

To know something, just as a youngster knows where the puzzle piece goes, is one thing. But to actually apply that knowledge and make the puzzle piece fit is another. Spiritual wisdom is the same way. We can *know* the Bible without putting it into practice—Satan proved that. To apply what we know in our daily walk is something we have to be intentional about. Take time to seek God's wisdom and understanding as you pursue His Kingdom today.

BREAKFAST:
Tofu Scramble Breakfast Bowl
(page 74)

LUNCH:
International Hummus Bowl
(page 106)

MIDDAY SNACK:
Buffalo Cauliflower Dip
(page 143) with veggies

DINNER:
Fava Bean and Mushroom
"Pot Roast" (page 130)

DAY 14

Therefore, as soon as they heard the sound of the horn, flute, zither, lyre, harp and all kinds of music, all the nations and peoples of every language fell down and worshiped the image of gold that King Nebuchadnezzar had set up.

DANIEL 3:7

An idol is anything we value more highly than God. This could be a favorite food, a sports team, a feeling of control—you name it! Hear me when I say that in and of themselves, these things are not bad. But when our love for these things loses its place, our trust in the Lord loses its place as well. You are now two weeks into the Daniel Fast. What has it been like to give up foods you value, even temporarily? As you continue on with this partial fast, remind yourself to worship the Creator, not the created. Trust the Lord to supply everything you need.

BREAKFAST:
Chickpea-Flax "Omelet"
with Spinach and Scallions
(page 72)

LUNCH:
Make-Ahead Quinoa Salad in
a Jar (page 90)

MIDDAY SNACK:
Buffalo Cauliflower Dip
(page 143) with veggies

DINNER:
Lemon-Artichoke Zucchini
Noodles (page 131) with
Chilled Tomato and Basil
Salad (page 91)

DAY 15

Behold, I stand at the door and knock. If anyone hears my voice and opens the door, I will come in to him and eat with him, and he with me.

REVELATION 3:20 (ESV)

Sometimes you just miss your family. I was having one of those weeks. I decided to take a spontaneous weekend road trip to visit my twin sister in Indianapolis. I set the surprise up with her roommates, and the plan was working perfectly. Parking my car, I had butterflies in my stomach. I knocked on the door. No answer. I checked—yes, I was at the right apartment. I knocked again . . . no answer. Finally, one of her roommates opened the door. Stepping in, I found my sister at the top of the steps, afraid of whoever was knocking on the apartment door so late in the evening. Of course, once she realized it was me, my plan was executed and memories were made. But that one moment of fearing the unknown caused a brief hold on what was in store. Is fear or unbelief holding you back from sitting at the table with the Creator? What would it look like to take one small step forward in faith today, knowing that He is the one who holds your life in His hands?

BREAKFAST:
Customizable Overnight Oats (page 68)

LUNCH:
Leftover Chilled Tomato and Basil Salad (page 91)

MIDDAY SNACK:
Fresh fruit

DINNER:
Roasted Chiles Rellenos with Cashew Cheese (page 132)

DAY 16

Now when Daniel learned that the decree had been published, he went home to his upstairs room where the windows opened toward Jerusalem. Three times a day he got down on his knees and prayed, giving thanks to his God, just as he had done before.

DANIEL 6:10

Because Daniel was the most distinguished high official of the king, those who ranked under him sought to find a complaint against him. Daniel, however, was found to be blameless. Because of this, the people presented an ordinance to the king that whoever would pray to anyone but the king for 30 days would be thrown into a den of lions. That's where this week's scripture picks up.

Daniel's commitment to the Lord was unshaken by this ordinance, and when the people saw him praying, they turned him in. But Daniel had confidence that his God would deliver—and did He ever! When Daniel was thrown in the lions' den, the mouths of the lions were shut, and he was delivered from certain death. Prayer creates a posture of humility and reverence toward the one true God. I pray that our faith would be rooted in this same foundation as we move forward, knowing that the same power that was used to shut the mouths of lions is alive in us today.

BREAKFAST:
Sweet Potato and Brussels Sprouts Hash (page 73)

LUNCH:
Asian-Style Stir-Fry Zoodle Bowl (page 97)

MIDDAY SNACK:
White Bean Hummus (page 141) with vegetables

DINNER:
Lemon-Artichoke Zucchini Noodles (page 131) with Roasted Vegetable Medley (page 138)

DAY 17

I am the vine; you are the branches. If you remain in me and I in you, you will bear much fruit; apart from me you can do nothing.

JOHN 15:5

When I think of this passage, I think about grapevines. Growing up, we had a winery attached to the back side of our property. We would walk to the edge of the woods and watch the growth process throughout the year. In order for these branches to grow and produce fruit, they must be attached to the vine.

To abide means to stay or to accept. What does Jesus mean when He says to remain in Him? In his book *Gospel*, J. D. Greear writes that abiding in the love of Christ means "feeling it, saturating ourselves with it, reflecting on it, standing in awe of it." But as we abide, our focus must be pointed not to the fruit, but to Christ alone. Greear sums it up beautifully when he says, "You concentrate on Jesus. You rest in His love and acceptance given to you not because of what you have earned, but because of what He has earned for you." Make your home in Christ and allow him to give you all of the nourishment you need to live the life He has purposed for you.

BREAKFAST:
Customizable Overnight Oats (page 68)

LUNCH:
Lentil Greek Salad (page 89)

MIDDAY SNACK:
Nuts and fruit

DINNER:
Quinoa and Black Bean Burger (page 111) with Roasted Mushrooms (page 136)

DAY 18

You are the light of the world. A town built on a hill cannot be hidden . . .
In the same way, let your light shine before others, that they may see your
good deeds and glorify your Father in heaven.

MATTHEW 5:14, 16

Once, when my niece and nephew were younger, I got them some glow-in-the-
dark pajamas. Even though it was still light out, they were so excited that they
put them on immediately, and we ran to the bathroom and closed the door. In the
darkness, we could see the glow from their pajamas, which caused the kind of gig-
gles that would melt any aunt into a puddle on the floor. What I loved about those
pajamas was that the glow was present in the darkness. As Christians, we are
called to be the light of the world. The light illuminates the dark, standing out as
it draws people to itself. This is what the gospel does to believers and why we are
called to a life of boldness. This light we have cannot be hidden, blending in with
the cultural expectations today. Pastor and writer Matt Damico said, "We won't
win the world by looking like it, or by fitting in, but by being different." Pray for
boldness in sharing the light that you have with the world around you, and when
the opportunity comes, let that light shine for the glory of the Lord.

BREAKFAST:
Fruit-Topped Chickpea Crepes
(page 71)

LUNCH:
Brown Rice, Mushroom, and
Kale Soup (page 81)

MIDDAY SNACK:
White Bean Hummus
(page 141) and vegetables

DINNER:
Lentil Shepherd's Pie
(page 126)

DAY 19

Brothers and sisters, I do not consider myself yet to have taken hold of it. But one thing I do: Forgetting what is behind and straining toward what is ahead, I press on toward the goal to win the prize for which God has called me heavenward in Christ Jesus.

PHILIPPIANS 3:13–14

In the 1992 Barcelona Olympics, Derek Redmond was set to run the 400-meter semifinal. He had proven himself as a prominent runner years before by breaking the British record in 1985. The gun went off, sending the athletes off the blocks and sprinting toward the finish line. However, at the 250-meter mark, Redmond went down, tearing a hamstring. Determined to finish, Derek started hobbling to the finish line. If you watch the video, you can see his father pushing through the crowd to get to his son and help him cross the finish line.

As believers, we are all running toward the eternal prize to which we have been called. There are moments in our race when we stumble and fall, but we have a Father who is willing to hold us up and walk with us through every situation that comes our way. Focusing on Him helps us realize that the things around us are small in comparison with this prize of eternity. Today, focus on the One who is willing to hold you up and give you the strength to keep pressing toward the promise of eternity with Him.

BREAKFAST:
Blueberry-Lemon Oatmeal Muffins (page 70)

LUNCH:
Vegetable Hash Bowl (page 104)

MIDDAY SNACK:
Leftover Brown Rice, Mushroom, and Kale Soup (page 81)

DINNER:
Spicy Vegetable-Stuffed Peppers (page 119) with Vegetarian Fried Cauliflower Rice (page 144)

DAY 20

Fight the good fight of the faith. Take hold of the eternal life to which you were called when you made your good confession in the presence of many witnesses.

1 TIMOTHY 6:12

If you've seen the first Captain America movie, you know that before he becomes part of the "super soldier" experiment that makes him a superhero, Chris Evans's character starts out as a guy so small and wormy that he can't even lie himself into the military. In an early scene, he gets into a fistfight with someone being disrespectful about the ongoing war effort. Even though he's no match for his opponent and he's hit to the ground several times, he stands up and says, "I could do this all day." Many times in life we feel beat down, unable to get up and move forward. However, the Bible encourages us to fight the good fight of faith because of the eternal promise we are called to in Jesus Christ. Paul also encourages us not to lose heart, because even if one's physical self is wasting away, one's inner self is being renewed day by day. Hold on to these promises as you take on today and remember that the difficulties you face are preparing you for an "eternal glory that far outweighs them all" (2 Corinthians 4:17).

BREAKFAST:
Customizable Overnight Oats
(page 68)

LUNCH:
Make-Ahead Quinoa Salad in
a Jar (page 90)

MIDDAY SNACK:
Carrot sticks and hummus

DINNER:
Mushroom Stroganoff with
Zucchini Ribbons (page 122)
and Chilled Tomato and Basil
Salad (page 91)

DAY 21

I ate no choice food; no meat or wine touched my lips; and I used no lotions at all until the three weeks were over.

DANIEL 10:3

Congratulations! The Lord has given you the strength to make it to this day. I know there were difficult moments, filled with temptation and desire for those things you love. However, the commitment you made to the Lord overshadowed those desires, and I pray that your relationship with Him has strengthened over the past three weeks. I want to encourage you to go back through your journal, look at your prayer board, and be reminded of how the Lord revealed Himself during this time. Making this commitment may not have been easy, but hopefully it was humbling to know that you stepped out in faith with a desire to draw closer to your Creator. My prayer for you is that you found a new strength, peace, and confidence in your relationship with the Lord and have a greater revelation of who He is. But don't stop here. Join a Bible study group or commit to serving at your church—keep digging.

Second Corinthians 8:9 says, "For you know the grace of our Lord Jesus Christ, that though he was rich, yet for your sake he became poor, so that you through his poverty might become rich." Reading this verse opened my eyes to the abounding grace and unconditional love He has extended to us. Although we cave to temptation, we can always be reminded that we have victory through salvation in Jesus Christ. In Him, we find inexpressible joy, peace, contentment, and hope that will last for eternity.

BREAKFAST:
Customizable Overnight Oats
(page 68)

LUNCH:
Vegan Faux Pho (page 84)

MIDDAY SNACK:
Granola Bites (page 69)
and fruit

DINNER:
Quinoa-Vegetable Stew
(page 129)

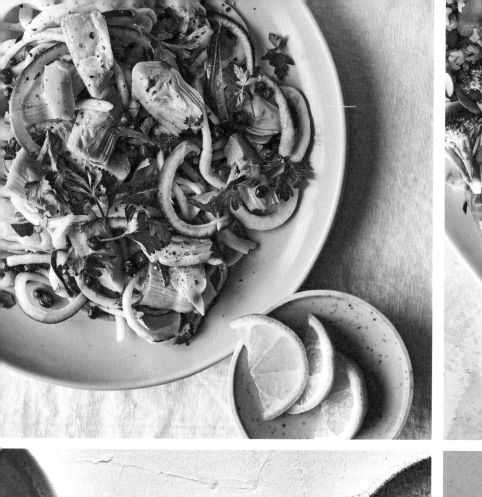
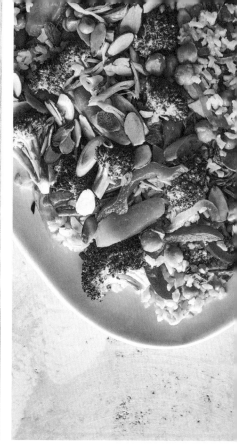
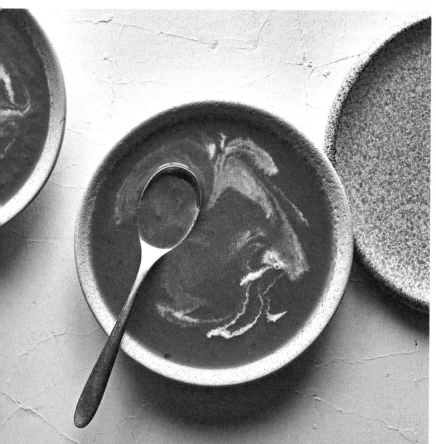
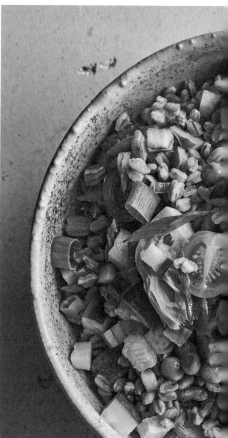

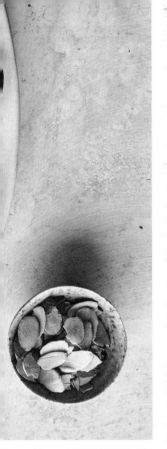

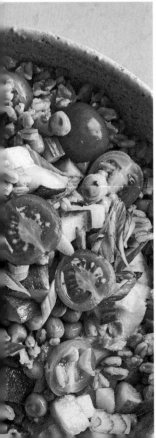

PART III

DANIEL FAST RECIPES

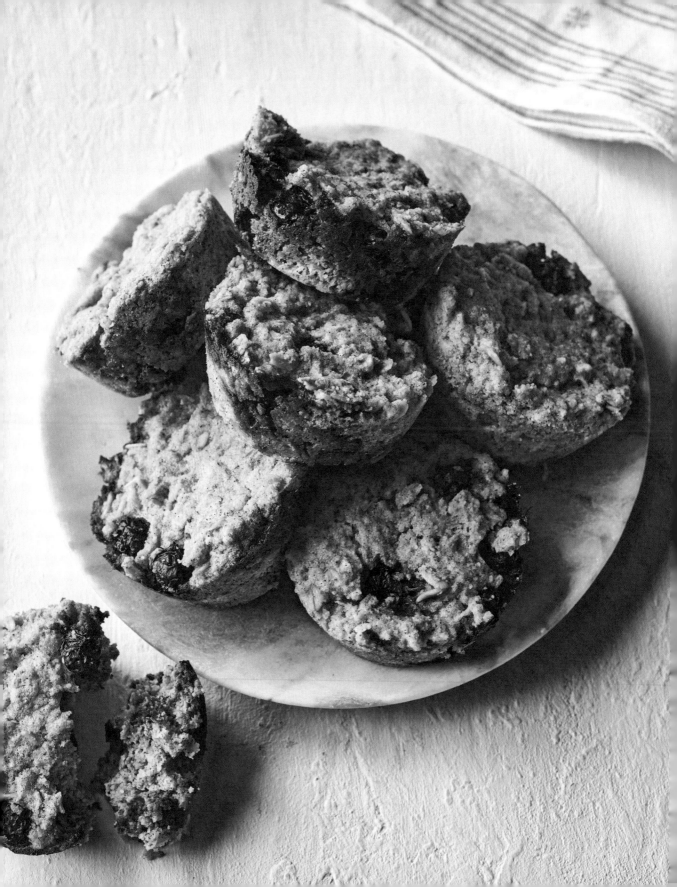

CHAPTER 5

Morning Morsels

‹ Blueberry-Lemon Oatmeal Muffins

Customizable Overnight Oats

SERVES 1 · PREP TIME: 5 MINUTES, PLUS AT LEAST 2 HOURS IN THE REFRIGERATOR

What could be better than waking up with breakfast already made? These overnight oats are customizable and easy to make. Simply give your oats a quick stir and let the toppings do the talking! This dish is ideal for meal prepping, as it stays good in the refrigerator for up to 5 days.

½ cup old-fashioned
   rolled oats
½ cup distilled water
1 tablespoon chia seeds
Desired toppings (e.g.,
   chopped nuts, banana
   slices, dried cranberries)

1. Stir together the oats, water, and chia seeds in a jar. Cover the jar and refrigerate it for at least 2 hours, preferably overnight.

2. When you're ready to eat, stir the contents of the jar, add toppings, and enjoy!

Granola Bites

MAKES 10 TO 12 BARS · PREP TIME: 10 MINUTES · COOK TIME: 10 MINUTES

Some breakfast dishes double as a midday snack, like these Granola Bites! Cut them larger for the 3 p.m. daily slump, or smaller for a quick breakfast on the go. They store great in a sealable container or bag for up to four days.

10 Medjool dates, pitted
1 cup raw unsalted almonds
3 tablespoons almond butter
1½ cups rolled oats
⅓ cup unsweetened shredded coconut

1. Preheat the oven to 350°F. Line a baking sheet with parchment paper.

2. Pulse the dates in the food processor until you see small pieces start to clump together. Set aside.

3. Lay the almonds in a single layer on the baking sheet. Bake for 10 to 12 minutes, or until they begin to slightly brown. Let them cool, then roughly chop. Keep the parchment paper on the baking sheet.

4. Warm the almond butter in a small saucepan over low heat.

5. In a large bowl, use a spatula to mix together the dates, chopped almonds, almond butter, rolled oats, and shredded coconut.

6. Pour the mixture onto the baking sheet and press down using your hands to evenly distribute.

7. Lifting with the parchment paper, bring the block of granola out off of the baking sheet and place it on a wooden cutting board.

8. Use a sharp chef's knife or pizza wheel to evenly cut the solid granola into squares.

Indeed, the very hairs of your head are all numbered. Don't be afraid; you are worth more than many sparrows.

LUKE 12:7

When I think of bites, I think of something small. Scripture tells us that even the smallest things are numbered by God. Remember today that He cares for you, even in the smallest parts of life.

Blueberry-Lemon Oatmeal Muffins

MAKES 12 MUFFINS • PREP TIME: 10 MINUTES • COOK TIME: 25 MINUTES

It took me a few tries to get this recipe just right following the Daniel Fast guidelines, but this combination gives the muffins a nice flavor—and makes the entire house smell amazing!

2 tablespoons
   flaxseed meal
6 tablespoons
   distilled water
1½ cups almond flour
1 cup old-fashioned
   rolled oats
1 teaspoon cinnamon
½ teaspoon kosher salt
¼ cup coconut oil, melted
   and cooled, plus more
Juice of 1 lemon (about
   2 tablespoons)
1 cup homemade almond
   milk (see tip)
1 teaspoon pure
   vanilla extract
1 cup fresh blueberries

1. Set a rack in the center of the oven. Preheat the oven to 350°F.

2. To make your flax eggs, whisk together the flaxseed meal and distilled water. Let sit for 5 to 15 minutes.

3. Brush 12 muffin cups with melted coconut oil.

4. In a large mixing bowl, whisk together the almond flour, rolled oats, cinnamon, and salt. Add the coconut oil, lemon juice, almond milk, flax eggs, and vanilla. Whisk until smooth.

5. Use a wooden spoon to fold in the blueberries.

6. Divide the batter among the muffin cups and bake for 22 to 25 minutes, or until an inserted toothpick comes out clean.

7. Let cool for 5 minutes. Then transfer the muffins to a wire rack until they're cool enough to enjoy.

TIP: Store-bought almond milk is not ideal on the Daniel Fast because it's processed in a factory. However, it's easy to make your own almond milk! Soak 1 cup of raw almonds overnight in cool water. Blend the soaked almonds with 4 to 5 cups of filtered water and ⅛ teaspoon salt until creamy. Then use a nut-milk bag or cheesecloth to strain the milk. Transfer to a covered bottle and store in the refrigerator for 4 to 5 days.

Fruit-Topped Chickpea Crepes

30-MINUTE MEAL

MAKES 4 CREPES · PREP TIME: 5 MINUTES · COOK TIME: 8 MINUTES

To stay gluten-free, these crepes are made with chickpea flour, which can be found in many grocery stores or ordered online. You can fill or top your crepe with any seasonal fruit, or even spread some almond butter on one side of the crepe and fold it over!

1¼ cups chickpea flour
1½ cups distilled
    water, divided
⅛ teaspoon kosher salt
2 tablespoons coconut oil
Fresh blueberries
Fresh strawberries, sliced
1 banana, sliced

1. In a blender on medium, puree the chickpea flour, 1 cup of water, and salt until smooth. With the blender on low, slowly pour in the distilled water until you have a thin batter.

2. Heat a crepe pan or sauté pan (about 10 inches in diameter) over medium-high heat. Let the pan get hot. Add ½ tablespoon of coconut oil and wait until the oil is completely melted and very hot.

3. Add ⅓ cup of batter to the pan in a circular motion, beginning from the center of the pan and moving outward, creating as thin a layer as possible. Then, grab the pan's handle and do a circling motion to let the batter spread evenly in the pan. Let cook for 2 minutes. Then flip over the crepe and cook for an additional 2 minutes.

4. To serve, top with the fresh fruit and roll the crepe up into a flute shape.

TIP: You can swap out the fruit for diced avocado, chopped tomato, chopped cucumber, and thinly sliced red onion for a more savory dish!

Chickpea-Flax "Omelet" with Spinach and Scallions

30-MINUTE MEAL

SERVES 1 · PREP TIME: 10 MINUTES · COOK TIME: 15 MINUTES

A traditional breakfast staple can easily be adapted to a gluten-free, plant-based form with the right ingredients. This protein-packed omelet features chickpea flour (available at many stores or online) and flaxseed meal as a fluffy and delicious substitute for eggs.

1 cup chickpea flour

2 tablespoons flaxseed meal

½ teaspoon kosher salt, plus more

½ teaspoon turmeric powder

1¼ cups distilled water, room temperature

2 tablespoons coconut oil, divided

1 garlic clove, finely chopped

1 shallot, finely chopped

4 cups baby spinach, packed

½ cup frozen petite peas

2 scallions, sliced

¼ teaspoon freshly ground black pepper

1. In a mixing bowl, whisk together the chickpea flour, flaxseed meal, ½ teaspoon of the salt, and turmeric. As you continue to whisk, slowly add the water until the mixture is smooth. Set the bowl aside.

2. Heat a large sauté pan over medium-high heat. Add the coconut oil to the pan, followed by the garlic and shallot. Cook for 2 minutes.

3. Add the spinach and toss around in the oil. Stir in the peas and scallions. Season with the salt and pepper. Cook for about 7 minutes. Remove the pan from the heat and set aside.

4. Heat a nonstick sauté pan over medium-high heat, then add the remaining tablespoon of coconut oil. Once the oil is hot, spoon the chickpea flour mixture into the pan. Grab the pan's handle and make a circular motion to evenly spread the batter over the entire pan.

5. Let the batter cook 2 to 3 minutes, until the bottom becomes golden brown. Then, carefully flip it over and cook for another 2 to 3 minutes. (Sliding the spatula around the edges as the omelet is cooking will help you monitor the cooking process on the bottom.)

6. Top one side with the spinach filling, and then fold over. Serve immediately.

Sweet Potato and Brussels Sprouts Hash

MAKE-AHEAD

SERVES 2 · PREP TIME: 10 MINUTES · COOK TIME: 45 MINUTES

I pray you won't miss the egg on top of this Daniel Fast hash! This recipe is full of flavor, but you can also crank up the heat with some chopped jalapeños and red pepper flakes. Even if you're cooking for one, this dish is great for leftovers and can even double as a side dish.

1 large sweet potato, washed, peeled, and cut into ½-inch cubes

3 to 4 tablespoons melted coconut oil, divided

½ pound Brussels sprouts, halved

½ yellow onion, chopped

1 red bell pepper, chopped

2 garlic cloves, chopped

1 teaspoon smoked paprika

1 teaspoon kosher salt

½ teaspoon freshly ground black pepper

½ teaspoon ground cumin

⅛ teaspoon cayenne pepper

1 small jalapeño pepper, seeded and chopped (optional)

¼ teaspoon red pepper flakes (optional)

1. Preheat the oven to 425°F. Line a baking sheet with parchment paper.

2. Lay the sweet potato cubes evenly over half of the baking sheet. Brush with 1 tablespoon of the melted coconut oil. Roast for 20 minutes.

3. Remove the baking sheet from the oven. Add the Brussels sprouts, onion, and bell pepper to the empty half of the baking sheet. Brush with 1 tablespoon of the melted coconut oil. Roast for an additional 15 minutes. (This means the sweet potatoes will roast for a total of 35 minutes.)

4. Heat 1 to 2 tablespoons coconut oil in a large cast-iron pan over medium-high heat. Add the garlic and stir. Toss in the roasted vegetables and season with the paprika, salt, pepper, cumin, cayenne pepper, jalapeño pepper (if using), and red pepper flakes (if using). Enjoy!

TIP: This is a great make-ahead to enjoy during the week. Store in individual serving containers and just reheat when you're ready to eat.

Tofu Scramble Breakfast Bowl

QUICK PREP

MAKES 2 BOWLS · PREP TIME: 5 MINUTES · COOK TIME: 8 MINUTES

Who needs eggs when tofu gives you all the richness you desire? As a vegan alternative to scrambled eggs, this dish for two is easily customizable for any breakfast craving. Here I use avocado with a sprinkle of fresh herbs, but you can let your creativity soar!

1 (8-ounce) package
  firm tofu
1 tablespoon coconut oil
6 cherry tomatoes, halved
2 scallions, sliced
½ teaspoon kosher salt
½ teaspoon freshly ground
  black pepper
¼ to ½ teaspoon turmeric
1 avocado, sliced
Fresh parsley or basil

1. In a mixing bowl, use a fork to crumble the tofu into small bite-size pieces.

2. Heat a large sauté pan over medium-high heat, then add the coconut oil. Once the oil is hot, add the tofu and tomatoes, and let cook for 5 to 8 minutes. Add the scallions. Then season with the salt, pepper, and turmeric.

3. To serve, divide the mixture into two bowls. Then top with the avocado slices and fresh parsley or basil.

TIP: Store any leftovers in an airtight container in the fridge for up to three days.

Sweet Potato Breakfast Muffins

MAKE-AHEAD, FREEZER-FRIENDLY

MAKES 12 MUFFINS • PREP TIME: 10 MINUTES • COOK TIME: 55 MINUTES

This recipe is inspired by egg muffins that are the perfect meal when you're on the go. There are a few steps to this recipe, but it makes 12 individual breakfast muffins to enjoy all week or freeze for later.

2 large sweet potatoes, sliced into very thin rounds
3 tablespoons coconut oil, divided
1¼ cup chickpea flour
2 cups distilled water, room temperature
1 shallot, finely chopped
1 bell pepper (any color), chopped
1 (12-ounce) bag baby spinach
1 teaspoon dried basil
1 teaspoon kosher salt
½ teaspoon freshly ground black pepper

1. Preheat the oven to 375°F. Line a baking sheet with parchment paper.

2. Arrange the sweet potato slices in an even layer on the baking sheet. Bake for 15 minutes or until they just begin to soften, then remove from the oven and set aside. Reduce the oven temperature to 350°F.

3. Melt 1½ tablespoons of coconut oil by microwaving it for 30 seconds. Then use the oil to brush 12 muffin tins. Line the sweet potato slices at the bottoms and around the sides of the muffin tins as tightly as possible. Set aside.

4. In a mixing bowl, whisk together the chickpea flour and water. Set aside.

5. Heat a sauté pan over medium heat. Heat the remaining 1½ tablespoons of coconut oil in the pan, then add the shallot and bell pepper. Cook for about 2 minutes, then add the spinach. Cook for another 2 minutes, then season with the basil, salt, and pepper.

6. Add the spinach mixture to the chickpea batter, then evenly fill each muffin tin. Bake for 30 minutes or until firm in the center.

7. Let cool for 5 minutes, then transfer the muffins to a wire rack until they're cool enough to enjoy.

Lemon Energy Pancakes

30-MINUTE MEAL

MAKES 12 PANCAKES · PREP TIME: 5 MINUTES, PLUS 15 MINUTES FOR FLAX EGGS TO SET
COOK TIME: 6 MINUTES PER PANCAKE

This recipe uses flax eggs instead of eggs and almond milk instead of milk. Since store-bought almond milk is processed in a factory, it's preferable to make your own in advance (see page 70). Top with fresh fruit, or cook fresh blueberries with 2 teaspoons of lemon juice in a small saucepan until it turns into a delicious and natural syrup!

2 tablespoons
  flaxseed meal
6 tablespoons
  distilled water,
  room temperature
2 cups almond flour
1 tablespoon chia seeds
¼ teaspoon kosher salt
2 tablespoons walnuts,
  chopped (optional)
1 tablespoon freshly
  squeezed lemon juice
2 cups homemade
  almond milk
Coconut oil

1. To make the flax eggs, whisk together the flaxseed meal and water. Set aside for 5 to 15 minutes.

2. In a large bowl, whisk together the almond flour, chia seeds, and salt. Add the walnuts (if using), lemon juice, almond milk, and flax eggs, and stir to combine.

3. Heat a griddle pan or large sauté pan over medium heat. Lightly coat with coconut oil.

4. For each pancake, pour about ¼ cup of batter. Cook for 2 to 3 minutes, until the edges begin to bubble. Then flip over the pancake and cook the other side for another 2 to 3 minutes or until golden brown. Repeat until you run out of batter.

> *For the kingdom of God is not a matter of eating and drinking, but of righteousness, peace and joy in the Holy Spirit.*
>
> ROMANS 14:17
>
> **Remember that just as the body is nourished with food, your spirit is nourished by the presence of your Creator. Find your strength in Him today.**

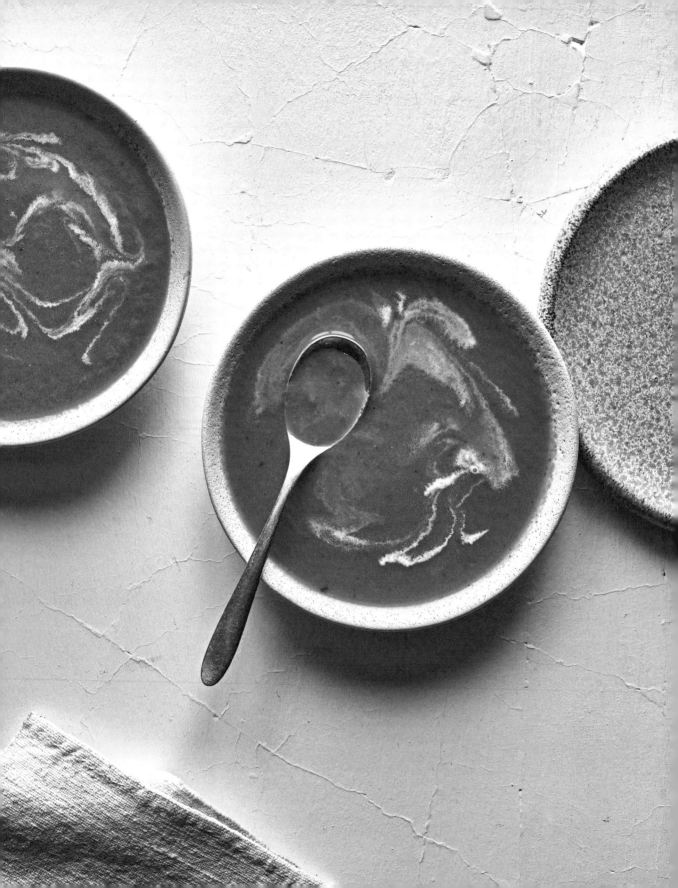

CHAPTER 6

Soups and Salads

< Roasted Tomato and Red Pepper Soup

Vegetable Soup with Basil Pesto

MAKE-AHEAD

SERVES 4 • PREP TIME: 20 MINUTES • COOK TIME: 20 MINUTES

Have you ever noticed how people's faces just light up when you say the word "pesto"? There's nothing like the smell of fresh basil pesto mingling with a rich, brothy soup full of nutritious veggies.

1 tablespoon olive oil

1 medium yellow or white onion, finely chopped

2 medium carrots, finely chopped

2 celery stalks, finely chopped

2 garlic cloves, minced

1 teaspoon dried thyme

1 teaspoon kosher salt

½ teaspoon freshly ground black pepper

6 cups low-sodium vegetable broth or stock

1 (15-ounce) can petite diced tomatoes with juices

2 zucchini, chopped

1 (15-ounce) can cannellini beans, drained and rinsed

½ cup Pesto with Walnuts (page 149), divided

1. Heat the oil in a Dutch oven or large stockpot over medium-high heat. Stir in the onion, carrots, and celery. Sauté the vegetables until tender, about 5 minutes.

2. Season with the garlic, thyme, salt, and pepper. Add the vegetable broth and diced tomatoes. Stir to combine.

3. Let the soup come to a light boil. Then lower the heat to medium and stir in the zucchini and cannellini beans. Cover and cook until heated through, about 10 minutes.

4. Add ¼ cup of the pesto into the soup and stir well.

5. To serve, ladle the soup into each bowl and top with a teaspoon of fresh pesto.

Brown Rice, Mushroom, and Kale Soup

SERVES 4 • PREP TIME: 15 MINUTES • COOK TIME: 30 MINUTES

Perfect for those chilly moments when you need a warm meal, this Brown Rice, Mushroom, and Kale Soup is sure to satisfy your savory cravings. And if you cook the rice ahead of time, you'll be surprised at how quickly this soup comes together!

1 cup brown rice, uncooked

3 tablespoons olive oil

1¼ pound cremini mushrooms

1 garlic clove, minced

2 tablespoons shallots, diced

1 teaspoon dried thyme

1 teaspoon dried cumin

1 teaspoon kosher salt

½ teaspoon freshly ground black pepper

½ teaspoon ground coriander

5 cups low-sodium vegetable broth

4 cups chopped kale

1. Cook the brown rice according to the package directions.

2. While the rice is cooking, heat the olive oil in a Dutch oven or large stockpot over medium heat. Add the mushrooms and sauté for about 7 minutes, stirring often.

3. Add the garlic and shallots, and sauté for 3 minutes while continuing to stir.

4. Add the thyme, cumin, salt, pepper, and coriander. Stir to combine.

5. Pour in the vegetable broth and bring to a light boil. Then stir in the kale and cook, covered, for 15 minutes.

6. Stir the cooked rice into the soup and let simmer for another 5 minutes. Serve hot.

Roasted Tomato and Red Pepper Soup

MAKE-AHEAD, FREEZER FRIENDLY

SERVES 4 • PREP TIME: 20 MINUTES • COOK TIME: 1 HOUR, 10 MINUTES

The combination of tomato and red peppers is just delicious. I always keep a can of coconut milk in my refrigerator, so when I make this soup, I just open the can, scoop out the solid top of the milk, and dollop or swirl it on the soup.

2½ pounds Roma tomatoes, halved

1½ teaspoons kosher salt, divided

1 teaspoon freshly ground black pepper, divided

2 tablespoons olive oil, divided

2 large red bell peppers, whole

1 small onion, diced

2 garlic cloves, chopped

1 teaspoon dried thyme

1 teaspoon dried basil

5 cups low-sodium vegetable broth, divided

1. Preheat oven to 400°F. Line two baking sheets with parchment paper.

2. Put the tomatoes in a large bowl and add 1 teaspoon of the salt, ½ teaspoon of the black pepper, and 1 tablespoon of the olive oil. Toss together. Then spread across one of the baking sheets in an even layer.

3. Lay the bell peppers on another baking sheet lined with parchment paper. Roast both vegetables for 40 minutes, flipping the bell peppers (but not the tomatoes) halfway through.

4. Remove both baking sheets from the oven and set the tomatoes aside. Put the peppers in a large bowl, cover it with plastic wrap, and let it sit for 10 minutes to loosen the peppers' skin.

5. When the peppers are cool enough to handle, remove the skins and chop.

6. Heat the remaining 1 tablespoon of olive oil in a Dutch oven or large stockpot over medium heat. Add the onion, garlic, thyme, basil, and the remaining ½ teaspoon salt and ½ teaspoon pepper. Sauté for 7 minutes, stirring occasionally.

7. Put the roasted tomatoes, roasted peppers, and onion mixture in a blender with 2 cups of the vegetable broth. Puree until smooth. (If your blender is small, you may have to do this in a few batches.)

8. Put the puree in the Dutch oven along with the remaining 3 cups of vegetable broth.

9. Stir, cover, and cook for 20 minutes at medium heat.

The name of the Lord is a fortified tower; the righteous run to it and are safe.

PROVERBS 18:10

When we seek comfort and strength in the things of this world, we will ultimately find emptiness and disappointment. Only in Christ will we find the strength and safety we need to fill our hearts' desires.

Vegan Faux Pho

SERVES 2 · PREP TIME: 30 MINUTES · COOK TIME: 1 HOUR

This recipe may seem like it has a long list of ingredients, but most of them are seasonings for the delicious broth. I tested out a lot of different spices to find the perfect blend, and this was the magic combination!

4 medium zucchini

1 teaspoon kosher salt

3 tablespoons olive oil, divided

1 large white onion, peeled and quartered

3-inch piece of fresh ginger, peeled and diced

4 star-anise pods

3 whole cloves

2 cinnamon sticks

2 cardamom pods

2 teaspoons whole coriander seeds

8 cups low-sodium vegetable stock

8 ounces shiitake mushrooms, thinly sliced

2 heads baby bok choy, halved

1 carrot, thinly sliced

1 cup broccoli florets

1 cup snow peas

½ cup bean sprouts

1 lime, quartered

2 scallions, sliced

1. Cut off the ends of the zucchini and turn them into zucchini noodles by using either a spiralizer or a vegetable peeler. Season with the salt, place in a colander, and let sit for 20 to 30 minutes.

2. Heat 1 tablespoon of the olive oil in a Dutch oven or large stockpot over medium-high heat. Add the onion and ginger and sauté for about 7 minutes, until they begin to char.

3. Lower the heat to medium. Then add the star anise, cloves, cinnamon sticks, cardamom pods, and coriander seeds. Stir for 2 to 3 minutes, until fragrant.

4. Add the vegetable stock and bring to a simmer. Cover and let cook for about 25 minutes.

5. Heat 1 tablespoon of the olive oil in a large sauté pan over medium-high heat. Add the mushrooms and sauté for 5 to 6 minutes, stirring occasionally. Remove the mushrooms from the pan and set aside.

6. Add the bok choy, carrot, and broccoli to the pan and cook for 7 to 8 minutes. Add the snow peas and cook for an additional 3 minutes.

7. Use a hand strainer to remove the onion, ginger, and whole spices from the pot of stock. Then add the mushrooms and all the sautéed vegetables (but not the zucchini noodles) to the vegetable stock.

8. In the same sauté pan, over medium-high heat, heat the remaining 1 tablespoon of olive oil. Once the pan is very hot, add the zucchini noodles and toss with tongs for 2 minutes.

9. To assemble your pho, ladle a serving of vegetable stock and vegetables into each bowl. Then add a heaping helping of zucchini noodles. Top with the bean sprouts, lime quarters, and scallions.

Hearty Tuscan Chili

MAKE-AHEAD, ONE-POT

SERVES 4 • PREP TIME: 20 MINUTES • COOK TIME: 30 MINUTES

My husband and I love Tuscany, and a few years ago we got the chance to take a cooking class there. We made so many great dishes, including a chili using fresh herbs from their garden. This is my take on that recipe. Feel free to substitute 2½ teaspoons of Italian seasoning for the individual herbs!

1 tablespoon coconut oil or olive oil

10 small red potatoes, cleaned and halved

1 medium yellow onion, finely chopped

2 garlic cloves, finely minced

1½ cup frozen corn

1 teaspoon dried thyme

1 teaspoon dried oregano

1 teaspoon dried parsley

1 teaspoon dried basil

1 teaspoon kosher salt

½ teaspoon freshly ground black pepper

½ teaspoon red pepper flakes

2 cups low-sodium vegetable stock

2 tablespoons tomato paste

2 (15-ounce) cans navy beans, drained and rinsed

1. Heat the oil in a Dutch oven or large stockpot over medium-high heat.

2. Add the potatoes and sauté for 7 to 9 minutes, stirring often. Add the onion and garlic, and sauté for 2 minutes, stirring often.

3. Stir in the corn, then season with the thyme, oregano, parsley, basil, salt, black pepper, and red pepper flakes.

4. Add the vegetable stock and tomato paste. Stir to combine, and bring to a high simmer.

5. Add the navy beans, cover, and reduce to a medium simmer. Let simmer for 10 minutes. Serve hot.

TIP: This is a perfect make-ahead dish when you're meal prepping for the week. You can store it in a sealed container in the refrigerator for up to 4 days.

Italian Chopped Salad

SERVES 2 • PREP TIME: 20 MINUTES

Chopped salads are a simple way to add variety to your day, and to use up ingredients you may not know what to do with. For a grab-and-go lunch, put all the ingredients in a jar, then add dressing and shake it up when you're ready to eat!

1 large head romaine, chopped
1 (15-ounce) can chickpeas, drained and rinsed
2 jarred roasted red peppers, chopped
1 carrot, chopped
1 celery stalk, chopped
6 artichoke hearts, quartered or chopped
8 cherry tomatoes, halved
1 cup cucumber, chopped
10 olives (any kind)
¼ cup thinly sliced red onion
2 to 4 tablespoons Green Goodness Dressing (page 148)
Fresh basil leaves, torn

1. In a large bowl, toss together the romaine, chickpeas, red peppers, carrot, celery, artichoke hearts, cherry tomatoes, cucumber, olives, red onion, and Green Goodness Dressing.

2. Before serving, top with the torn basil leaves.

Power Greens with Roasted Butternut Squash

SERVES 2 · PREP TIME: 20 MINUTES · COOK TIME: 35 MINUTES

Some people eat butternut squash only in the fall or winter, but it can be delicious all year round. This simple but flavorful salad is great comfort food for cold days, without being too heavy for a summer dinner. Try the squash alone with the dressing, or mashed with sea salt and olive oil.

1 (3-pound) butternut squash, peeled and cubed

1½ tablespoons olive oil, plus more

1 teaspoon kosher salt, plus more

½ teaspoon freshly ground black pepper, plus more

¼ cup raw pecans

2 cups baby spinach

1 cup baby kale

3 tablespoons dried cranberries

2 to 4 tablespoons Homestyle Italian Herb Dressing (page 151)

1. Position a rack in the center of the oven and preheat the oven to 425°F. Line a large baking sheet with parchment paper.

2. In a large bowl, toss the butternut squash cubes in the olive oil, salt, and pepper. Spread the squash across the baking sheet in a single layer. Roast for 30 minutes, or until fork tender, flipping the cubes with a spatula halfway through. Set aside.

3. Heat a large sauté pan over medium heat. Toast the pecans in the pan for 1 to 2 minutes. (Be sure to stay at the stove, as they can burn fast!) Remove the pecans from the pan and set aside.

4. In a large bowl, toss together the spinach, kale, and dried cranberries. Drizzle half of the dressing over the mixture. Then top with the butternut squash and toasted pecans. Drizzle the rest of the dressing on top and serve.

Lentil Greek Salad

SERVES 2 · PREP TIME: 20 MINUTES · COOK TIME: 15 MINUTES

Why are we using French lentils in a Greek salad? They're small, they don't get mushy easily, and they have a nutty, peppery flavor that pairs well with the rest of the salad's ingredients. But if you can't find French lentils, any lentils will do.

1 cup uncooked petite French lentils, rinsed and sorted
3 cups packed baby spinach
½ cup thinly sliced red onion
½ cup chopped cucumber
½ cup kalamata olives, pitted and quartered
12 cherry tomatoes, halved
⅓ cup fresh flat-leaf parsley, chopped
¼ cup extra-virgin olive oil
2 tablespoons red wine vinegar
1 garlic clove, minced
1 teaspoon dried oregano
½ teaspoon sea salt
¼ teaspoon freshly ground black pepper

1. Cook the lentils according to the package directions. Drain any extra liquid.

2. In a large salad bowl or serving platter, put the spinach on the bottom, followed by the cooked lentils. Top with the red onion, cucumber, olives, tomatoes, and parsley.

3. In a small bowl, whisk together the olive oil, vinegar, garlic, oregano, salt, and pepper. (I also like to put all the dressing ingredients in a canning jar, cover, and shake.)

4. Pour the dressing over the salad and serve. (Don't toss, or you'll lose the beautiful layers!)

Beloved, I urge you as sojourners and exiles to abstain from the passions of the flesh, which wage war against your soul.

1 PETER 2:11 (ESV)

There are moments when temptations seem sweeter than wholehearted surrender to our Creator. Allow Him to equip you with the weapons to fight these temptations through prayer, fasting, and time in His Word. Seek His face today.

Make-Ahead Quinoa Salad in a Jar

MAKE-AHEAD

MAKES 2 QUART-SIZED SALADS · PREP TIME: 20 MINUTES · COOK TIME: 15 MINUTES

Quinoa, a nutritional powerhouse, adds extra texture and an earthy flavor to this salad, while hearty vegetables keep it fresh and crunchy. I like to use Homestyle Italian Herb Dressing, but you can try out any dressing you like!

1 cup uncooked quinoa, rinsed

¾ cup thinly chopped red cabbage

1 cup baby kale

1 large carrot, chopped or shredded

1 cucumber, chopped

¼ cup thinly sliced red onion

½ cup frozen petite peas

6 cherry tomatoes, halved

2 to 4 tablespoons Homestyle Italian Herb Dressing (page 151)

1. Cook the quinoa according to the package directions. Let cool in a bowl.

2. Place a layer of red cabbage at the bottoms of 2 mason jars. Then add a layer of baby kale to each jar. Continue creating layers with the carrot, cucumber, red onion, peas, and cherry tomatoes. (The frozen peas will have thawed by the time you eat the salad.)

3. When you're ready to eat, add 1 to 2 tablespoons of dressing to your jar, shake, and enjoy!

Chilled Tomato and Basil Salad

QUICK PREP

SERVES 2 · PREP TIME: 5 MINUTES, PLUS 30 MINUTES TO CHILL

When I was a little girl, my grandparents had a large garden. Every dinner, my Nana would make a tomato and basil salad. It's so easy and truly great with any dish or just by itself.

1 pint of cherry
  tomatoes, halved
10 to 12 basil leaves
3 tablespoons extra-virgin
  olive oil
1 teaspoon sea salt

1. Toss the cherry tomatoes and basil together in a bowl and refrigerate for 30 minutes.

2. Drizzle with the olive oil and season with salt. Stir gently and serve immediately!

Consider it pure joy, my brothers and sisters, whenever you face trials of many kinds, because you know that the testing of your faith produces perseverance. Let perseverance finish its work so that you may be mature and complete, not lacking anything.

JAMES 1:2–4

We are not called to live lives of comfort but lives that are wholly surrendered to our Creator. In doing so, He will develop us into who He calls us to be, making us complete in all that He is. Trust His process as you walk through this day.

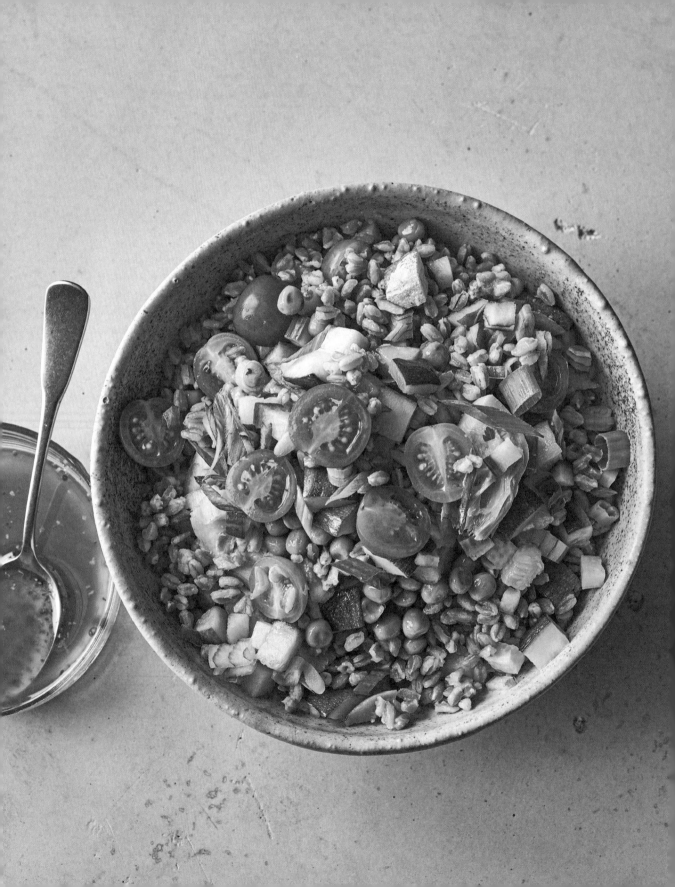

Buildable Bowls

< Italian Farro Bowl

Roasted Vegetable Power Bowl

MAKE-AHEAD

MAKES 2 BOWLS • PREP TIME: 10 MINUTES • COOK TIME: 40 MINUTES

If I'm going to turn on my oven to roast vegetables, then I'm going to be efficient and roast as many vegetables as I can! This bowl is perfect for using up leftover roasted vegetables from the week, which warm up so nicely after a few minutes in the oven.

1 small butternut squash, cubed (about 2 cups)

1½ tablespoons olive oil, divided

1½ teaspoons kosher salt, divided

1 teaspoon garlic powder

1 teaspoon onion powder

½ teaspoon cumin

1 cup broccoli florets

¼ teaspoon freshly ground black pepper

½ red bell pepper, thinly sliced

4 packed cups chopped baby kale

½ cup black beans, rinsed and drained

⅓ cup raw walnuts

1 avocado, halved and sliced

2 to 4 tablespoons Green Goodness Dressing (page 148)

1. Preheat the oven to 400°F. Line two large baking sheets with parchment paper.

2. In a large bowl, toss the butternut squash cubes with 1 tablespoon of the olive oil, 1 teaspoon of the salt, the garlic powder, the onion powder, and the cumin. Spread them across one of the baking sheets and roast 20 to 25 minutes, until golden brown and fork tender.

3. Toss the broccoli in a bowl. Then add in ½ tablespoon olive oil, ½ teaspoon salt, and black pepper. Add the broccoli and the bell pepper to the other baking sheet in a single layer. Roast for 15 minutes.

4. To assemble the bowls, divide the kale and put a layer of it at the bottom of each bowl. Then add the butternut squash, broccoli, bell pepper, and black beans.

5. Top each bowl with walnuts, avocado slices, and 1 to 2 tablespoons of Green Goodness Dressing. Enjoy!

TIP: For a lighter dressing, whisk together a bit of extra-virgin olive oil, a squeeze of lemon juice, and a dash of salt and pepper.

Italian Farro Bowl

MAKES 2 BOWLS · PREP TIME: 10 MINUTES · COOK TIME: 30 MINUTES

Farro is truly one of the most versatile grains. It's hearty and goes with almost any dish, warm or cold. I normally cook up an entire package of farro at once and use it in different dishes throughout the week.

1 cup uncooked farro

1 tablespoon extra-virgin olive oil

1 large zucchini, chopped

¼ teaspoon kosher salt

⅛ teaspoon freshly ground black pepper

1 cup cucumber, seeded and finely chopped

6 artichoke hearts, quartered

12 cherry tomatoes, halved

1 cup petite peas

¼ cup chopped red onion

2 scallions, thinly sliced

2 to 4 tablespoons Homestyle Italian Herb Dressing (page 151)

1. Cook the farro according to the package directions. Then set aside.

2. Heat the olive oil in a sauté pan over medium-high heat. Add the zucchini, season it with salt and pepper, and sauté for 7 minutes, stirring frequently. Set the pan aside.

3. To assemble the bowls, divide up the farro between both bowls.

4. Equally divide the zucchini, cucumber, artichoke hearts, cherry tomatoes, and peas on top of the farro.

5. Sprinkle the red onion and scallions over the top.

6. Drizzle 1 to 2 tablespoons of Homestyle Italian Herb Dressing on top of each bowl.

7. Toss together and enjoy!

TIP: *When using grains during the week, cook up the entire package and divide it into amounts you will need for other meals. This will cut down on your cooking time. Cooked grains will keep for 5 days refrigerated in a sealed container.*

Fiesta Rice Bowl with Tofu

MAKES 2 BOWLS • PREP TIME: 30 MINUTES • COOK TIME: 20 MINUTES

Mexican-inspired dishes are so much fun! Everyone gets excited when I tell my family we're eating Mexican food tonight. This dish is sure to become a favorite during your Daniel Fast and beyond!

1 cup uncooked brown rice
1 (12-ounce) package extra-firm tofu
2 tablespoons olive oil, divided, plus more for finishing
1 yellow or white onion, chopped
1 bell pepper (any color), chopped
1 tomato, chopped
1 jalapeño pepper, seeded and diced
1 garlic clove, minced
½ teaspoon kosher salt
½ teaspoon chili powder
½ teaspoon paprika
½ teaspoon cayenne pepper
¼ teaspoon freshly ground black pepper
1¼ cup finely shredded cabbage (or any greens)
1 (15-ounce) can black beans, drained and rinsed
1 lime, halved
1 avocado, mashed
Fresh cilantro

1. Cook the brown rice according to the package directions.

2. To prepare the tofu, lay a few paper towels on a plate or other clean work surface, set the tofu on top, and then put several more paper towels on top of the tofu. Place a heavy pan or other heavy item on top of the paper towels and let it sit for at least 10 minutes or up to 30 minutes. (This presses the moisture out of the tofu so it can absorb more flavor when you cook it.) Cut the tofu into ½-inch cubes.

3. Heat 1 tablespoon of the olive oil in a large sauté pan over medium heat. Sauté the onion and bell pepper for 2 minutes. Add the tomato, jalapeño, garlic, salt, chili powder, paprika, cayenne pepper, and black pepper. Cook for 5 minutes. Then remove the pan from the heat and transfer the mixture of vegetables to a bowl.

4. Heat the remaining 1 tablespoon of olive oil in the sauté pan until it's very hot. Add the tofu and cook for 8 to 10 minutes or until golden brown, flipping the cubes over halfway through.

5. To assemble the bowls, divide the cabbage in half and create a layer at the bottom of each bowl. Divide the cooked rice and create a heap in the middle of each bowl. Then surround the edges with the cooked vegetables. Top one side with the tofu and the other side with the black beans.

6. To finish off the bowls, squeeze a lime half over each bowl, drizzle with olive oil, and top with the avocado and cilantro.

Asian-Style Stir-Fry Zoodle Bowl

MAKES 2 BOWLS • PREP TIME: 30 MINUTES • COOK TIME: 15 MINUTES

I grew up on pasta and noodles. We also had zucchini at nearly every meal. So zucchini noodles, also known as "zoodles," are a natural fit for me! They're so easy to prepare, and if you don't have the time to spiralize them yourself, you can buy them prepared in most grocery stores.

1 (12-ounce) package extra-firm tofu

2 large zucchini, spiralized (or peeled into "zoodles")

1 teaspoon kosher salt, divided

1 tablespoon coconut oil or olive oil, plus more

1 red bell pepper, thinly sliced

1 cup fresh snow peas

1¼ cup shredded red cabbage

1 cup shredded carrots

¼ cup microgreens or live sprouts

2 scallions, thinly sliced

Handful chopped cilantro

1 lime, quartered

Extra-virgin olive oil or avocado oil, for finishing

1. To prepare the tofu, lay a few paper towels on a plate or other clean work surface, set the tofu on top, and then put several more paper towels on top of the tofu. Place a heavy pan or other heavy item on top of the paper towels and let it sit for at least 10 minutes or up to 30 minutes. (This presses the moisture out of the tofu so it can absorb more flavor when you cook it.) Cut the tofu into ½-inch cubes.

2. Put the zucchini noodles in a colander and season with ½ teaspoon of the salt. Cover with a paper towel and let it sit for 20 minutes. (This removes liquid from the zucchini and gives you a crispier zoodle.)

3. Heat the oil in a large sauté pan over medium-high heat. Carefully add the tofu cubes and cook for 4 to 5 minutes. Then flip them over and cook them for an additional 4 to 5 minutes, or until they're golden brown. Transfer the tofu cubes to a bowl or dish.

4. Add the bell pepper and snow peas to the same pan. Season with the remaining ½ teaspoon of salt, and sauté for 3 minutes. Remove from heat.

5. To assemble the bowls, divide the zoodles between two bowls. Top each bowl with the tofu cubes, bell pepper, snow peas, red cabbage, carrots, microgreens, scallions, and cilantro.

6. Squeeze the juice of one lime wedge over each bowl. Then drizzle olive oil or avocado oil on top. Serve the bowls warm.

Crispy Cauliflower Super Bowl

MAKES 2 BOWLS • PREP TIME: 15 MINUTES, PLUS OVERNIGHT FOR THE MUSHROOMS TO SOAK
COOK TIME: 30 MINUTES

Tapioca flour is a gluten-free way to create a nice crisp texture on the cauliflower in this recipe. I'm also substituting dried mushrooms for soy sauce, since most soy sauce contains gluten. Soaking the mushrooms overnight and then pureeing them gives this dish a deep, rich flavor.

¼ ounce dried mushrooms
1 cup warm water
2 tablespoons kosher salt, plus ½ teaspoon
1 head cauliflower, chopped into florets
¼ cup coconut oil, plus 1 tablespoon
2 cups tapioca flour, plus 2 teaspoons
¼ cup vegetable broth or stock
1 teaspoon unseasoned rice vinegar
1 teaspoon red pepper flakes
1 garlic clove, minced
1 teaspoon minced fresh ginger
1 red bell pepper, sliced
1 zucchini, chopped
¼ teaspoon freshly ground black pepper
2 scallions, thinly sliced
2 teaspoons toasted sesame seeds

1. In a small bowl, put the dried mushrooms in the warm water. Let them soak overnight. Discard the water, rinse the mushrooms, and puree them in a blender. Set them aside.

2. Bring a large pot of water to a boil. Add 2 tablespoons of the salt. Then add the cauliflower florets. Boil the florets for 2 minutes. Then drain the florets and transfer them to a bowl of ice water. Let them sit in the ice bath for 5 minutes, then drain and transfer to a large plate.

3. Heat ¼ cup of the coconut oil in a large skillet or cast-iron pan over medium-high heat. Let the oil get very hot.

4. Put 2 cups of the tapioca flour in a bowl. Coat the cauliflower florets in the tapioca flour. Then carefully add the florets to the pan of oil. Fry the florets for 8 to 10 minutes, or until lightly browned. Then transfer the fried florets to a dish lined with paper towels. Repeat in batches until all the florets are fried.

5. In a large sauté pan or skillet over medium heat, whisk together the vegetable broth, rice vinegar, pureed mushrooms, red pepper flakes, garlic, and ginger. Keep whisking as you slowly add the remaining 2 teaspoons of tapioca flour until the sauce thickens.

6. Add the crispy cauliflower florets to the pan of sauce and gently toss to coat. Reduce the heat and keep warm.

7. Wipe out the pan you used to fry the cauliflower florets. Add 1 tablespoon of coconut oil to the pan. Heat the oil over medium-high heat. Add the bell pepper and zucchini, and season them with the remaining ½ teaspoon of salt and the black pepper. Cook for about 7 minutes, then remove the pan from the heat.

8. To assemble your bowl, divide the peppers and zucchini between two bowls. Top each bowl with the crispy cauliflower florets. Garnish with the scallions and sesame seeds.

For we have no power to face this vast army that is attacking us. We do not know what to do, but our eyes are on you.

2 CHRONICLES 20:12

As you walk through today, remember that He is fighting for you. Fix your gaze on Him and allow Him to soften your heart to what He has for you as you continue through this journey.

Quinoa Veggie Bowl

MAKES 2 BOWLS · PREP TIME: 15 MINUTES · COOK TIME: 45 MINUTES

I love all of the vegetables and flavors in this dish, and I hope you enjoy them as well. Feel free to add or swap in seasonal vegetables you have available in your area.

1 cup uncooked quinoa, rinsed

1 medium head of cauliflower, cut into florets

5½ tablespoons extra-virgin olive oil, divided

1 teaspoon ground cumin

½ teaspoon ground coriander

½ teaspoon turmeric

½ teaspoon kosher salt, plus more

¼ teaspoon freshly ground black pepper, plus more

1 zucchini, chopped

1 red cabbage thinly sliced

1 red onion, thinly sliced

2 tablespoons apple cider vinegar

1 cup baby kale

Juice of 1 lemon

1 (15-ounce) can chickpeas, rinsed and drained

1. Cook the quinoa according to the package instructions.

2. Preheat the oven to 400°F. Line two baking sheets with parchment paper.

3. In a medium bowl, toss the cauliflower florets in 2 tablespoons of olive oil. Add the cumin, coriander, turmeric, ½ teaspoon salt, and ¼ teaspoon pepper. Toss to thoroughly coat.

4. Spread the cauliflower florets in an even layer on one of the prepared baking sheets. Roast the florets for 30 minutes. Remove them from the baking sheet and put them in a bowl. Set the bowl aside.

5. Toss the zucchini with 1 tablespoon of olive oil and season lightly with salt and pepper. Put the zucchini on the second baking sheet and roast it for 13 minutes.

6. In a large bowl, toss together the cabbage, red onion, apple cider vinegar, and 2 tablespoons of olive oil.

7. In a separate bowl, toss the baby kale with the lemon juice until thoroughly coated.

8. To serve, divide up the quinoa and add it to one-quarter of each bowl, followed by a scoop each of cauliflower florets, zucchini, and chickpeas. Place a handful of kale in the middle of the bowl. Then top with red cabbage and red onion.

9. Drizzle ½ tablespoon of extra-virgin olive oil over each bowl and serve.

Green Goodness Superfood Bowl with Avocado

30-MINUTE MEAL

MAKES 2 BOWLS · PREP TIME: 10 TO 30 MINUTES

This bowl is full of fresh vegetables, with the avocado and dressing adding a creamy texture. Try adding 1 cup of quinoa or brown rice to each bowl if you want a heartier meal.

1 medium zucchini
2 cups baby spinach
1 cup shaved red cabbage
1 green apple, spiralized
  or chopped
1 cup shelled edamame,
  steamed or boiled
1 avocado, halved
  and sliced
1 cup pea shoot sprouts
  or microgreens
2 scallions, thinly sliced
2 to 4 tablespoons Green
  Goodness Dressing
  (page 148)

1. Cut off both ends of the zucchini and either spiralize it or create ribbons using a vegetable peeler. Put the zucchini noodles in a colander and let them sit for 10 to 30 minutes.

2. To assemble the bowls, divide the zucchini noodles between two bowls. In each bowl, add 1 cup of baby spinach over the zucchini, followed by the cabbage, apple, and edamame.

3. Top each bowl with avocado slices, pea shoot sprouts or microgreens, and scallions. Finish each bowl with 1 to 2 tablespoons of Green Goodness Dressing.

Because your steadfast love is better than life, my lips will praise you.

PSALM 63:3 (ESV)

Allow worship and praise to overwhelm you today, knowing that His love is better than life itself.

Crunchy Nut and Quinoa Bowl

MAKES 2 BOWLS • PREP TIME: 15 MINUTES • COOK TIME: 20 MINUTES

The protein-packed combination of quinoa and nuts makes this bowl a perfect dinner at the end of a long day. Nuts add texture and a rich flavor to the quinoa, and the dressing brings out the bright flavor of the fresh vegetables.

1 cup uncooked quinoa, rinsed

3 tablespoons almonds

3 tablespoons cashews

2 tablespoons sesame seeds

2 tablespoons pepitas

1 cup baby kale

1 cup shredded green or red cabbage

1 carrot, grated

½ (15-ounce) can chickpeas, drained and rinsed

½ red bell pepper, diced

¼ cup diced red onion

2 scallions, thinly sliced

2 to 4 tablespoons Homestyle Italian Herb Dressing (page 151)

1. Cook the quinoa according to the package directions. Set aside.

2. Heat a sauté pan over medium-low heat. In batches, place the almonds, cashews, sesame seeds, and pepitas in the pan. Toast for 30 seconds to 1 minute. Then set aside.

3. To assemble, divide the quinoa between two bowls. Then add the kale, cabbage, carrot, chickpeas, bell pepper, and red onion. Top with the toasted nuts and seeds as well as the scallions. Finish each bowl with 1 to 2 tablespoons of Homestyle Italian Herb Dressing.

Brussels Sprouts Slaw and Chickpea Bowl

MAKES 2 BOWLS · PREP TIME: 20 MINUTES · COOK TIME: 30 MINUTES

This bowl is super easy and quick to make yet full of flavor, especially if you buy pre-shaved Brussels sprouts at the store. (The shredding disk in your food processor also works great for this.) The combination of the chickpeas, apple, and almonds with the shaved Brussels sprouts makes a perfect meal.

½ (15-ounce) can chickpeas, drained and rinsed

1 pound fresh Brussels sprouts, shaved or shredded

1 apple, thinly sliced

3 tablespoons Dijon Vinaigrette (page 152)

3 tablespoons sliced almonds

1. Preheat the oven to 350°F. Line a baking sheet pan with parchment paper.

2. Pat the chickpeas dry with a paper towel. Spread them in an even layer on the sheet pan and bake for 30 minutes.

3. In a large bowl, combine the Brussels sprouts and sliced apple. Add the Dijon Vinaigrette and toss to coat.

4. To assemble the bowls, divide the Brussels sprouts mixture between the two bowls. Top each bowl with roasted chickpeas and sliced almonds. Serve immediately.

Vegetable Hash Bowl

MAKES 4 BOWLS · PREP TIME: 15 MINUTES · COOK TIME: 30 MINUTES

A hash packed with vegetables is the ultimate comfort food. This versatile and affordable dish is perfect for breakfast and dinner alike. Simply toss in your leftover vegetables, and this dish will quickly become a family favorite.

3 tablespoons coconut oil
1 pound small red or yellow
   potatoes, halved
1 medium sweet potato,
   chopped (skin on)
1 teaspoon Italian
   seasoning
1 teaspoon kosher salt
¼ teaspoon freshly ground
   black pepper
¼ teaspoon red
   pepper flakes
2 garlic cloves, minced
1 shallot, finely chopped
½ head broccoli, cut
   into florets
1 (8-ounce) package baby
   bella mushrooms, sliced
1 red or orange bell
   pepper, chopped
3 cups baby kale
Fresh parsley, chopped,
   for garnish
Extra-virgin olive oil,
   for garnish

1. Heat the coconut oil in a large sauté pan or cast-iron pan over medium-high heat. Add the potatoes and sweet potatoes, and cook for 12 minutes, flipping often, until browned on all sides.

2. Season with the Italian seasoning, salt, pepper, and red pepper flakes.

3. Add the garlic and shallot. Then add the broccoli florets and cook for 5 minutes, stirring frequently.

4. Add the baby bella mushrooms, bell pepper, and baby kale. Continue cooking for an additional 10 minutes.

5. To serve, divide the hash among four bowls. Top each bowl with fresh parsley and a drizzle of olive oil.

Truly he is my rock and my salvation; he is my fortress, I will not be shaken.

PSALM 62:6

Have you ever felt like this? So many days I find myself feeling shaken or "rocked." Find your strength in the God of your salvation—your fortress that will not be shaken.

Peanut-Lime Rice Bowl

MAKES 4 BOWLS · PREP TIME: 20 MINUTES · COOK TIME: 30 MINUTES

This bowl is bursting with complex flavor, and the smooth peanut butter adds a creamy, mellow finish. (Just make sure the peanut butter is all-natural to adhere to the fast!) It's delicious and filling just the way it is, but feel free to add some tofu or edamame for extra protein.

2 cups brown rice
½ cup smooth all-natural peanut butter
1 garlic clove, grated or crushed
2 tablespoons freshly squeezed lime juice
1 tablespoon fresh ginger, grated
¼ teaspoon red pepper flakes
2 teaspoons toasted sesame oil
2 cups baby kale
1 cup shaved red or green cabbage
1 red bell pepper, thinly sliced
4 scallions, thinly sliced
Fresh cilantro leaves, chopped
½ cup peanuts, roughly chopped

1. Cook the brown rice according to the package instructions.

2. In a mixing bowl, whisk together the peanut butter, garlic, lime juice, ginger, red pepper flakes, and sesame oil until smooth. If the mixture is too thick, whisk in 1 teaspoon of water at a time until you reach the desired consistency.

3. Toss the rice in the peanut dressing.

4. To assemble the bowls, divide the baby kale and the rice between four bowls, putting the kale on one side of the bowl and the rice on the other. Top with the cabbage, red bell pepper, scallions, fresh cilantro, and peanuts. Enjoy!

International Hummus Bowl

30-MINUTE MEAL

MAKES 2 BOWLS · PREP TIME: 10 MINUTES · COOK TIME: 15 MINUTES

Once assembled, this dish is as beautiful as it is delicious! The layers of color and texture create a share-worthy display, all while delivering the flavors you crave. It's portioned for two, so grab a friend for a lunch date to remember.

½ cup uncooked quinoa, rinsed

½ (15-ounce) can chickpeas, drained and rinsed

1 teaspoon extra-virgin olive oil

¼ teaspoon dried basil

¼ teaspoon dried oregano

¼ teaspoon garlic powder

2 cups greens (baby kale, spinach, or romaine lettuce)

¾ cup chopped cucumber

½ bell pepper, chopped

12 pitted kalamata olives

6 grape or cherry tomatoes, halved

½ cup White Bean Hummus (page 141)

2 to 4 tablespoons Homestyle Italian Herb Dressing (page 151)

1. Cook the quinoa according to the package directions.

2. Put the chickpeas in a medium bowl. Then add the olive oil and season with basil, oregano, and garlic powder. Stir to coat the chickpeas.

3. To assemble, divide the quinoa and the greens between two bowls. In their own quarters of the bowl, on top of the greens, add the cucumber, bell pepper, olives, and tomatoes.

4. Top with the chickpeas and a dollop of hummus in the center of each bowl. Drizzle with 1 to 2 tablespoons of dressing and enjoy!

TIP: You can use store-bought hummus as long as it's all-natural.

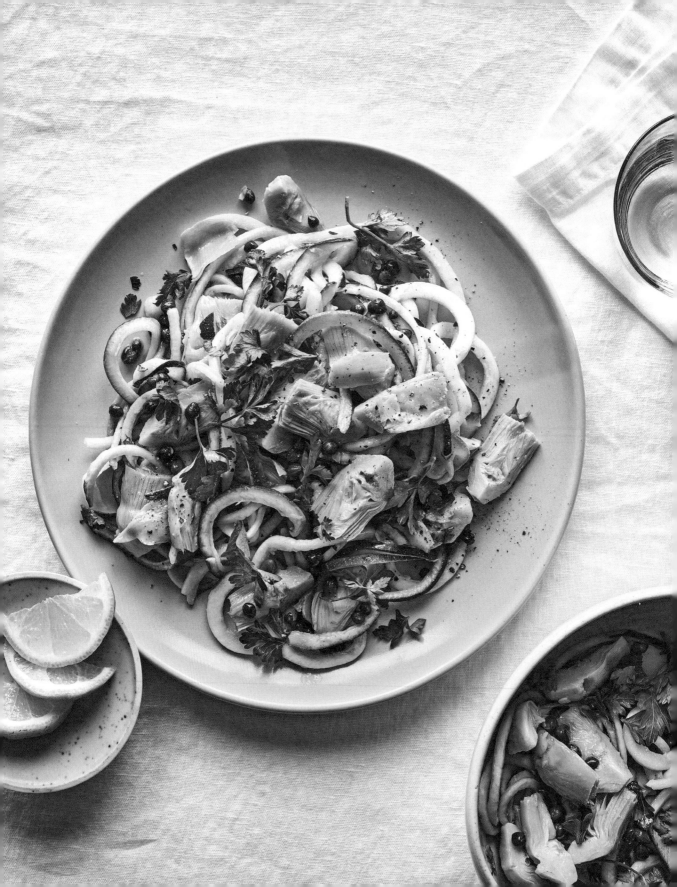

Meatless Mains

< Lemon-Artichoke Zucchini Noodles

Ginger-Sesame Vegetable Stir-Fry

30-MINUTE MEAL

SERVES 4 • PREP TIME: 15 MINUTES • COOK TIME: 15 MINUTES

The ginger in this recipe gives immense flavor to a surprisingly light dish. Don't forget to toast the almonds—when paired with the sesame oil, they create a truly memorable bite!

½ cup sliced almonds
1 tablespoon coconut oil
4 cups fresh broccoli florets
½ pound fresh green beans, cut in half
2 carrots, peeled and sliced
1 bell pepper (red or yellow), sliced
¾ cup thinly sliced red onion
1 teaspoon kosher salt
½ teaspoon freshly ground black pepper
2 garlic cloves, minced
1 teaspoon freshly grated ginger
4 cups baby kale
1 cup frozen petite peas
1 (15-ounce) can chickpeas, drained and rinsed
3 cups cooked brown rice
3 scallions, thinly sliced
1 tablespoon sesame oil

1. Put the almonds in a small sauté pan over medium heat. Toast for about 3 minutes, then remove the pan from the heat and set aside.

2. Heat the coconut oil in a large sauté pan or wok over medium-high heat. Add the broccoli florets, green beans, carrots, bell pepper, red onion, salt, and pepper. Sauté for 7 to 9 minutes, stirring occasionally.

3. Add the garlic, ginger, baby kale, peas, and chickpeas. Sauté for 3 to 4 minutes, stirring frequently.

4. Add the cooked brown rice and stir until combined with the vegetables. Stir in the scallions and then the sesame oil. Serve topped with the toasted almonds.

My grace is sufficient for you, for my power is made perfect in weakness.

2 CORINTHIANS 12:9

His grace will sustain you. Rest in this truth as you start to pray today.

Quinoa and Black Bean Burger

FREEZER-FRIENDLY

MAKES 6 BURGERS · PREP TIME: 20 MINUTES · COOK TIME: 10 MINUTES

This burger recipe is flavorful and filling. For a finer consistency (and extra quick prep), use a food processor to pulse the vegetables instead of finely chopping them. This is also a great recipe to double and freeze to eat later.

2 (15-ounce) cans black beans, drained and rinsed
1 cup cooked quinoa
½ cup finely chopped yellow onion
½ cup finely chopped bell pepper
1 jalapeño pepper, seeded and finely chopped (optional)
2 tablespoons chickpea flour
1 garlic clove, minced
1 teaspoon paprika
1 teaspoon kosher salt
½ teaspoon freshly ground black pepper
½ teaspoon cumin
½ teaspoon chili powder
⅛ teaspoon red pepper flakes
1½ tablespoons olive oil or coconut oil

1. In a large bowl, use a fork to mash some of the beans into smaller pieces. Add the quinoa, onion, bell pepper, jalapeño pepper (if using), chickpea flour, garlic, paprika, salt, pepper, cumin, chili powder, and red pepper flakes. Combine to form an even mixture. (If the mixture seems a little dry, add 1 tablespoon of water.)

2. Divide the mixture into 6 equally sized balls. Then flatten the balls to create burger patties.

3. Heat the oil in a large pan or indoor grill over medium-high heat. Then add the formed burger patties. Cook each side for about 4 minutes.

4. Serve over a salad or as a side dish.

Eggplant-Wrapped Veggie "Meat Loaf"

MAKE-AHEAD

SERVES 4 · PREP TIME: 35 MINUTES · COOK TIME: 1 HOUR, 30 MINUTES

Who knew you'd be begging for more meat loaf during the Daniel Fast? Okay, so it's actually made of lentils, but it's just as tasty as the real thing, and you'll be sure to get your veggies in with this one!

1 large eggplant
1 tablespoon flaxseed meal
3 tablespoons water
1 cup dry lentils, rinsed
    and sorted
2½ cups low-sodium
    vegetable broth
1 tablespoon coconut oil or
    olive oil
½ cup diced onion
½ cup diced red
    bell pepper
1 carrot, grated
1 celery stalk, diced
3 garlic cloves, minced
1 cup organic rolled
    oats, divided
1 tablespoon chopped
    fresh parsley
1 teaspoon dried thyme
1 teaspoon dried basil
1 teaspoon onion powder
1 teaspoon kosher salt,
    plus more
½ teaspoon freshly ground
    black pepper
½ to 1 cup Cashew Gravy
    (page 155) or Simple
    Marinara Sauce
    (page 154)

1. Cut off the ends of the eggplant and slice it lengthwise into 12 long, thin slices.

2. Make a layer of paper towels on a plate or cutting board and place a layer of eggplant slices on top of it. Cover with another layer of paper towels and add the remaining eggplant slices. Cover that with a final layer of paper towels and place another plate or cutting board on top. Let sit for 20 to 30 minutes, until the slices are relatively dry.

3. Make a flax egg by combining the flaxseed meal and water in a small bowl. Stir together and let sit for 5 to 15 minutes, until the texture is thick and egglike.

4. Put the lentils and vegetable broth in a large pot. Bring to a boil, reduce the heat to low, and simmer, covered, for about 35 minutes, stirring occasionally. Remove the lid and set the pot aside.

5. While the lentils are cooking, preheat the oven to 350°F and line a loaf pan with parchment paper.

6. Heat the oil in a large sauté pan over medium-high heat. Add the onion, bell pepper, carrot, celery, and garlic. Cook for about 5 minutes, stirring occasionally, until the onions and garlic are soft and fragrant.

7. In a large bowl, combine the cooked lentils, flax egg, and sautéed vegetable mixture. Stir together.

8. Stir ½ cup of the oats into the bowl. Take the remaining ½ cup of oats and pulse it in your food processor or blender until it has the consistency of flour. Stir this oat "flour" into the bowl as well.

9. Stir the parsley, thyme, basil, onion powder, salt, and pepper into the bowl.

10. Lightly season the eggplant with salt. Place two slices lengthwise down the center of the loaf pan. Then lay the rest of the slices crosswise, with their ends hanging over either side of the pan.

11. Transfer the loaf mixture from the bowl into the pan over the eggplant slices. Take the overhanging edges of the eggplant slices and fold them over the loaf pan so that it's now completely wrapped in eggplant slices.

12. Bake for 50 minutes.

13. Slice and serve, topped with Cashew Gravy or Simple Marinara Sauce.

TIP: Prepare this recipe a night or two before you want to eat it. Refrigerate it, and then bake when you're ready to enjoy.

Italian Lentil "Meatballs"

FREEZER-FRIENDLY

SERVES 4 · PREP TIME: 15 MINUTES · COOK TIME: 25 MINUTES

These Italian Lentil "Meatballs" are packed with garlic and a lot of flavor. They pair beautifully with Simple Marinara Sauce (page 154). Serve over zucchini noodles or put them on top of your salad. They go quick, so double the batch and freeze half to have on hand for another great Daniel Fast dish.

1 tablespoon flaxseed meal
2½ tablespoons
 distilled water
1 tablespoon olive oil or
 coconut oil
1 small onion, chopped
3 garlic cloves, chopped
2 cups cooked
 lentils, divided
½ cup almond meal
1 tablespoon chopped
 fresh parsley
1 teaspoon kosher salt
½ teaspoon freshly ground
 black pepper
½ teaspoon dried thyme
½ teaspoon dried basil
¼ teaspoon red
 pepper flakes

1. Preheat the oven to 400°F. Line a baking sheet with parchment paper.

2. In a small bowl, combine the flaxseed meal and water. Let sit for 5 to 15 minutes. This is your flax egg.

3. Heat the oil in a sauté pan over medium heat. Add the onion and garlic, and sauté for 2 to 3 minutes. Remove the pan from the heat and transfer the mixture to a food processor or blender. Pulse until finely chopped.

4. Add 1 cup of the lentils to the food processor, along with the flax egg, almond meal, fresh parsley, salt, pepper, thyme, basil, and red pepper flakes.

5. Transfer the mixture into a bowl with the remaining lentils and stir to combine.

6. Use a melon scoop or small ice cream scoop to create "meatballs." Place the formed balls on the baking sheet. Bake for 20 minutes.

The steadfast love of the Lord never ceases; his mercies never come to an end; they are new every morning; great is your faithfulness.

LAMENTATIONS 3:22-23 (ESV)

His mercies are new every single day. No matter what yesterday looked like or what tomorrow holds, rest in the present moment of His grace for you today.

Mushroom Ragù with Zucchini Noodles

MAKE-AHEAD

SERVES 4 • PREP TIME: 20 MINUTES • COOK TIME: 40 MINUTES

Bring new life to zucchini noodles with this mushroom ragù! Baby bella mushrooms, tomatoes, and Italian spices marry together to create this warm and inviting dish, ideal for family-style dinners.

3 to 4 medium zucchini
5 tablespoons olive
    oil, divided
1 medium yellow
    onion, diced
1 (12-ounce) package baby
    bella mushrooms,
    chopped
3 garlic cloves, finely
    chopped (divided)
1 teaspoon kosher salt
½ teaspoon freshly ground
    black pepper
1½ teaspoons dried
    oregano
1 teaspoon dried thyme
1 teaspoon dried sage
1 teaspoon dried rosemary
1 (32-ounce) can
    chopped tomatoes or
    crushed tomatoes
1 (6-ounce) can
    tomato paste

1. Cut the ends off the zucchini and turn them into zucchini noodles, either by using a spiralizer on the ribbon setting or by using a vegetable peeler. Season the zucchini noodles with a pinch of salt and put them in a colander covered with a paper towel for 20 minutes.

2. Heat a large skillet over medium heat. Once hot, add 2 tablespoons of olive oil and the onion. Sauté for 5 to 7 minutes, stirring often. Remove the onion with a slotted spoon and transfer onto a plate.

3. Add another 2 tablespoons of olive oil to the same skillet over medium-high heat.

4. Add the mushrooms and stir to coat in the oil. Add in 2 of the chopped garlic cloves, the salt, and the pepper. Sauté for about 5 minutes, stirring often.

5. Add the oregano, thyme, sage, rosemary, and sautéed onions, followed by the can of tomatoes. Stir again and bring to a boil.

6. Add the tomato paste, using your tablespoon or wooden spoon to press the paste along the edges of the pan to incorporate it into the sauce. To get any remaining tomato paste out of the can, fill the can with hot water, stir with a teaspoon, and pour into the sauce.

7. Reduce the heat and simmer, covered, for 15 to 20 minutes.

8. Heat a large sauté pan over medium heat. Add in the remaining 1 tablespoon of oil and the remaining garlic. Add the zucchini noodles and toss them around while cooking for 5 minutes.

9. Serve topped with the mushroom ragù.

Indian-Style Spicy Chickpeas

SERVES 4 • PREP TIME: 20 MINUTES • COOK TIME: 30 MINUTES

Grab your Dutch oven and get ready for your home to smell amazing. This chickpea dish is loaded with flavor and is sure to bring your taste buds to a new destination. Ladle each bowl thoughtfully and garnish with some fresh scallions for a beautiful presentation.

2 tablespoons coconut oil

1 medium onion, chopped

3 garlic cloves, chopped

1 jalapeño pepper, chopped

1 teaspoon freshly grated ginger

2 teaspoons ground cumin

2 teaspoons ground coriander

1 teaspoon curry powder

1 teaspoon kosher salt

¾ teaspoon cayenne pepper

½ teaspoon freshly ground black pepper

2 (15-ounce) cans chickpeas, drained and rinsed

2 (15-ounce) cans petite diced tomatoes (no salt added)

3 scallions, thinly sliced

1. Heat the coconut oil in a large Dutch oven or stockpot over medium-high heat.

2. Add the onion and sauté for 3 minutes. Add the garlic, jalapeño pepper, and ginger. Sauté for 2 minutes.

3. Season with the cumin, coriander, curry powder, salt, cayenne pepper, and black pepper. Stir to combine.

4. Add the chickpeas and petite diced tomatoes (including the juices). Stir together. Then cover the Dutch oven, reduce the heat to medium-low, and simmer for 25 minutes.

5. To serve, ladle a serving of chickpeas into each bowl and garnish with the scallions.

And let us run with perseverance the race marked out for us, fixing our eyes on Jesus, the pioneer and perfecter of faith. For the joy set before him he endured the cross, scorning its shame, and sat down at the right hand of God.

HEBREWS 12:1–2

Remember that set before Jesus was the cross, yet He humbly pursued it for you and me. Lay aside the things that keep you from running into His arms today as you prepare to encounter Him like never before.

Mediterranean Casserole

MAKE-AHEAD, ONE-POT

SERVES 4 · PREP TIME: 20 MINUTES · COOK TIME: 40 MINUTES

I love one-pot dishes! This one is filled with all your favorite vegetables, making it an easy win for the Daniel Fast. The flavors are complex, but the cleanup is simple!

2 tablespoons coconut oil or olive oil

1 medium butternut squash, cubed

2 yellow squash or zucchini, sliced

1 (12-ounce) package cherry tomatoes, halved

1 (12-ounce) package whole baby bella mushrooms

1 bell pepper, sliced

2 (15-ounce) cans petite diced tomatoes (no salt added)

1 teaspoon kosher salt

1 teaspoon oregano

1 teaspoon thyme

1 bay leaf

½ teaspoon freshly ground black pepper

½ teaspoon red pepper flakes

1 (15-ounce) can white beans

Fresh parsley for garnish

1. Preheat the oven to 350°F.

2. Heat a large braising pan or oven-proof skillet with a cover over medium-high heat.

3. Add the oil, followed by the butternut squash. Sauté for 7 minutes. Add the zucchini, cherry tomatoes, whole baby bella mushrooms, and bell pepper. Stir together and cook for 5 minutes.

4. Add the petite diced tomatoes (including the juices), followed by the salt, oregano, thyme, bay leaf, black pepper, and red pepper flakes.

5. Cover and put in the oven for 25 minutes.

6. Remove from the oven and add the white beans. Then return the pan to the oven for 5 minutes.

7. Serve garnished with fresh parsley.

Very Veggie Layer Lasagna

FREEZER-FRIENDLY

SERVES 4 • PREP TIME: 20 MINUTES, PLUS AT LEAST 2 HOURS FOR CASHEWS TO SOAK
COOK TIME: 1 HOUR, 10 MINUTES

Growing up in my Italian Nana's kitchen meant we had lasagna on Sundays. We also had meatballs and spaghetti, but we all loved her lasagna. Now you can enjoy a Daniel Fast–friendly version of it as well.

1½ cups raw cashews
½ cup distilled water
Juice of 1 lemon
1 to 2 garlic cloves, chopped
1 teaspoon dried oregano
½ teaspoon onion powder
½ teaspoon kosher salt, plus more
¼ teaspoon freshly ground black pepper, plus more
8 basil leaves
1 tablespoon coconut oil
1 (12-ounce) container mushrooms, sliced (any kind)
4 cups Simple Marinara Sauce (page 154)
4 medium zucchini, thinly sliced (using a mandoline or chef's knife)

1. Soak the raw cashews in water for at least 2 hours.

2. Preheat the oven to 350°F.

3. To make the "ricotta," drain the cashews and put them in a blender with the distilled water, lemon juice, garlic, oregano, onion powder, salt, pepper, and basil leaves. Blend until creamy. Transfer the "ricotta" into a bowl and refrigerate until ready to use.

4. Heat the coconut oil in a sauté pan over medium heat. Add the mushrooms and sauté for 7 minutes. Remove from heat.

5. Ladle enough marinara sauce into a 9-by-13-inch baking dish so that it covers the bottom in an even layer. Over the marinara sauce, create an even layer of zucchini slices, then a layer of "ricotta," and finally a layer of mushrooms. Repeat the layers again: marinara sauce, zucchini, "ricotta," and mushrooms. End with a final layer of zucchini and then marinara sauce.

6. Cover the baking dish with aluminum foil and bake for 45 minutes. Then uncover it and bake for an additional 15 minutes.

7. Let lasagna cool for 10 minutes before slicing and serving.

TIP: You can cut this lasagna up into squares and freeze individual portions in an airtight container.

Spicy Vegetable-Stuffed Peppers

MAKE-AHEAD

SERVES 4 · PREP TIME: 20 MINUTES · COOK TIME: 45 MINUTES

You can't go wrong with stuffed peppers! Packed with cauliflower rice and sweet potatoes, these peppers will leave you feeling full without the guilt. Prepped and cooked in about an hour, this dish will easily become a staple in your dinner rotation, Daniel Fast or no.

1 tablespoon olive oil

½ onion, chopped

1 sweet potato, peeled and chopped into small cubes

3 poblano peppers, diced

3 garlic cloves, chopped

1 (10-ounce) can diced tomatoes with green chiles

1 (8-ounce) bag frozen cauliflower rice

1 teaspoon cumin

1 teaspoon dried oregano

1 teaspoon kosher salt

½ teaspoon freshly ground black pepper

4 large green bell peppers

1. Preheat the oven to 375°F. Prepare a baking sheet by lining it with parchment paper.

2. To prepare the filling, heat the olive oil in a large sauté pan over medium heat. Add the onion, sweet potato cubes, poblanos, and garlic. Cook for 5 minutes, stirring occasionally.

3. Add the diced tomatoes with green chiles, cauliflower rice, cumin, oregano, salt, and pepper. Cover the pan, reduce the heat, and simmer for 10 minutes.

4. While the filling is simmering, cut the tops off the bell peppers—but don't discard them! Keeping the bell peppers intact, use a small knife to cut out the cores and seeds. Discard the cores and seeds. Place the hollow peppers on the baking sheet.

5. Once the filling is done, divide it into fourths and use it to fill the 4 peppers. Put the tops back on the peppers and bake for 30 minutes.

TIP: To make these stuffed peppers a little heartier, add in any leftover quinoa or lentils from earlier in the week.

Cauliflower Curry with Chickpea Pancakes

SERVES 2 · PREP TIME: 20 MINUTES · COOK TIME: 30 MINUTES

Chickpeas give a power-packed punch of protein, vitamins, and minerals with each serving, so I decided to make them a feature in this spiced-to-perfection dish. Use the pancakes as a vessel to scoop up the cauliflower curry.

FOR THE CAULIFLOWER CURRY

2 tablespoons coconut oil

1 head cauliflower, cut into bite-size florets

1 onion, chopped

2 garlic cloves, minced

1 (15-ounce) can petite diced tomatoes (no salt added)

2 cups vegetable broth

1 (15-ounce) can chickpeas, drained and rinsed

2 tablespoons curry powder

1 teaspoon thyme

1 teaspoon allspice

1 teaspoon cumin

1 teaspoon smoked paprika

1 teaspoon kosher salt

¾ teaspoon cayenne powder

½ teaspoon white pepper

2 scallions, thinly sliced

Fresh parsley

TO MAKE THE CAULIFLOWER CURRY

1. Heat the coconut oil in a large braising pan over medium-high heat. Add the cauliflower florets and cook for 3 minutes. Add the onion and garlic, and cook for another 4 minutes, stirring often.

2. Add the petite diced tomatoes, vegetable broth, chickpeas, curry powder, thyme, allspice, cumin, smoked paprika, salt, cayenne powder, and white pepper. Stir together and bring to a simmer.

3. Reduce the heat to medium, cover, and simmer for 15 minutes. Before serving, add the scallions and fresh parsley.

FOR THE CHICKPEA PANCAKES

1 cup chickpea flour
1½ cups distilled water
½ teaspoon kosher salt
¼ teaspoon freshly ground
   black pepper
¼ teaspoon turmeric
¼ teaspoon cumin
2 tablespoons coconut oil

TO MAKE THE CHICKPEA PANCAKES

4. Put the chickpea flour in a large mixing bowl and slowly whisk in the distilled water. Add the salt, pepper, turmeric, and cumin. Whisk until you have a smooth batter.

5. Heat a large sauté pan over medium-high heat. Add 1 tablespoon of the oil, and once it's very hot, pour in about ¼ cup of batter for each pancake. Aim for 3 or 4 mini pancakes per batch.

6. Cook the pancakes for 2 to 3 minutes. Then flip the pancakes and cook for another 1 to 2 minutes, or until golden brown.

7. Add more oil and cook a second batch of pancakes in the same way. If you still have batter left, cook a third batch. Serve with the cauliflower curry.

Mushroom Stroganoff with Zucchini Ribbons

SERVES 2 · PREP TIME: 30 MINUTES, PLUS 2 HOURS TO SOAK CASHEWS
COOK TIME: 20 MINUTES

This is a fresh twist on a normally heavy dish. Aside from the prep time it takes to soak the cashews, it's a quick trip from the stove to the table—and you can save even more time by making the sauce the night before.

1 cup raw cashews
2 to 3 medium zucchini
2 garlic cloves, minced
6 basil leaves
1 teaspoon dried parsley
1 teaspoon dried thyme
1 tablespoon freshly
 squeezed lemon juice
1 cup distilled water
½ teaspoon kosher salt
¼ teaspoon freshly ground
 black pepper
1 tablespoon coconut oil or
 olive oil
3 cups mushrooms, sliced

1. Soak the raw cashews in water for at least 2 hours.

2. Cut the ends off the zucchini and turn them into ribbons, either by using a spiralizer on the ribbon setting or by using a vegetable peeler. Season the zucchini noodles with a pinch of salt and put them in a colander covered with a paper towel for 20 minutes. (This removes the moisture.)

3. To make the sauce, drain the soaked cashews and put them in a blender or food processor with the basil leaves, parsley, thyme, lemon juice, water, salt, and pepper. Blend until smooth.

4. Heat the oil in a large sauté pan over medium-high heat. Sauté the mushrooms and garlic for 7 minutes.

5. Add the sauce to the pan and cook the mushrooms in it for 5 minutes, stirring often.

6. Add the zucchini ribbons, tossing with tongs to combine. Cover and let cook for 5 minutes before serving.

Mediterranean Vegetables
over Spaghetti Squash

MAKES 2 SERVINGS · PREP TIME: 30 MINUTES · COOK TIME: 1 HOUR, 10 MINUTES

Spaghetti squash has become very popular as a no-carb pasta option. I love how it takes on flavors from the foods around it. The first time I made this dish was for friends at church, and everyone loved it so much that there were no leftovers!

1 whole spaghetti squash
1 medium onion, thinly sliced
2 bell peppers (any color), thinly sliced
1 (12-ounce) container mushrooms (whole or sliced)
1 to 2 zucchini, cut into rounds
3 tablespoons olive oil, divided
1½ teaspoons dried thyme, divided
1½ teaspoons dried oregano, divided
1 teaspoon kosher salt, divided
½ teaspoon freshly ground black pepper
½ teaspoon red pepper flakes (optional)
Fresh herbs, chopped, for garnish

1. Preheat the oven to 425°F. Line two baking sheets with parchment paper or aluminum foil. Bake the spaghetti squash on one of the baking sheets for 45 minutes.

2. In a large bowl, toss the onion, bell peppers, mushrooms, and zucchini with 2 tablespoons of olive oil, 1 teaspoon of thyme, 1 teaspoon of oregano, ¾ teaspoon of salt, the black pepper, and the red pepper flakes (if using).

3. Spread the vegetables in an even layer on the other baking sheet. Roast for 25 minutes, flipping the vegetables with a spatula halfway through.

4. Remove the spaghetti squash and let cool for 10 minutes. When it's cool enough to handle, use a sharp chef's knife on a wooden cutting board to cut the squash in half. Use a spoon to remove the seeds and top layer of flesh. Then use a fork to remove the spaghetti strands.

5. Put the squash strands in a large serving bowl. Drizzle the remaining 1 tablespoon of olive oil over the strands. Then season with the remaining ½ teaspoon of thyme, ½ teaspoon of oregano, and ¼ teaspoon of salt. Toss to coat.

6. Top with the roasted vegetables. Serve garnished with fresh herbs.

Portabella Mushrooms with Cashew Ricotta

MAKE-AHEAD

MAKES 4 · PREP TIME: 10 MINUTES, PLUS 2 HOURS TO SOAK CASHEWS
COOK TIME: 20 MINUTES

As an Italian, I consider ricotta a staple. It's great by itself, over toast with jelly, on top of meatballs, and with mushrooms. Real ricotta isn't allowed on the Daniel Fast, but this cashew "ricotta" makes a great substitute. And a dollop of pesto gives the dish a vibrant color!

1½ cups raw cashews
½ cup distilled water
Juice of 1 lemon
2 garlic cloves,
    chopped, divided
1 teaspoon dried oregano
1 teaspoon kosher
    salt, divided
½ teaspoon freshly ground
    black pepper, divided
½ teaspoon onion powder
4 large portabella
    mushroom caps
20 basil leaves
½ cup extra-virgin olive oil

1. Soak the raw cashews in water for at least 2 hours. Drain them and put them in a blender or food processor with the distilled water, lemon juice, 1 chopped garlic clove, oregano, ½ teaspoon salt, ¼ teaspoon pepper, and the onion powder. Blend until creamy, then transfer to a bowl and set aside until ready to use.

2. Preheat the oven to 350°F. Prepare a baking sheet by lining it with parchment paper.

3. Clean the portabella mushrooms by lightly wiping the caps with a damp paper towel. Then flip them over, cut off the stems, and use a teaspoon to scoop out the gills.

4. Lightly brush the mushrooms with olive oil. Place them on the prepared baking sheet and bake for 12 minutes, or until golden brown.

5. Fill each mushroom cap with the cashew "ricotta" and put them back in the oven for another 10 minutes.

6. To make the pesto, put the basil leaves and olive oil in a blender or food processor, with the remaining salt, pepper, and garlic. Blend until you have the pesto consistency you desire.

7. Top each mushroom with a dollop of pesto before serving!

Vegetable-Hummus Collard Wrap

30-MINUTE MEAL

MAKES 2 WRAPS · PREP TIME: 20 MINUTES · COOK TIME: 1 MINUTE

Craving a burrito for your next Daniel Fast meal? This wrap satisfies your cravings in a healthy and flavor-filled way! The hummus holds all of the fresh flavors together while the microgreens add the perfect crunch.

2 leaves collard greens
½ cup White Bean
    Hummus (page 141)
1 small zucchini, cut into
    thin rounds or spiralized
1 to 2 carrots, grated
1 tomato, thinly sliced
1 avocado, halved, pitted,
    and sliced
Live sprouts
    or microgreens

1. To blanch the collard leaves, fill a large sauté pan with about 1 inch of water and bring it to a boil. Set a bowl of ice water next to it. Add each leaf to the boiling water for 30 seconds. Then use tongs to transfer the leaf immediately into the ice water. Let the leaf sit in the ice for 1 minute and then transfer it to a paper towel to dry.

2. Cut off the stems and lay both the leaves on a cutting board or other clean work surface.

3. Add a layer of hummus starting from the center of the leaf and going out, leaving about ¼ inch of the edge of the leaf showing. Then add the zucchini, carrots, tomato slices, and avocado. Top with sprouts or microgreens.

4. To fold, bring the two sides in toward the stem. Then roll up the leaf from the top down, as if you were rolling up a burrito. Leave the seam side down, cut in half, and enjoy!

Therefore, accept each other just as Christ has accepted you so that God will be given glory.

ROMANS 15:7 (NLT)

Have you ever asked yourself, "Does God accept me?" The answer is simple! Yes! He loves you so much, and He doesn't want sin in your life. Pray like a warrior during this Daniel Fast and lean on God to turn away from sin.

Lentil Shepherd's Pie

FREEZER-FRIENDLY, MAKE-AHEAD

SERVES 4 • PREP TIME: 15 MINUTES • COOK TIME: 1 HOUR

Whenever I want comfort food, shepherd's pie is my go-to! This was the first recipe I made the first time I did the Daniel Fast, and I loved it so much that I always make it this way now.

1 tablespoon olive oil, plus more

1 cup dry lentils (any color), rinsed and sorted

2 garlic cloves, minced

4 cups low- or no-sodium vegetable stock

1 bay leaf

1 teaspoon dried thyme

3 tablespoons tomato paste

2 tablespoons tapioca flour

2 tablespoons distilled water

1 (10-ounce) bag frozen mixed vegetables

1 teaspoon kosher salt, plus more

½ teaspoon freshly ground black pepper, plus more

2 pounds Yukon gold potatoes, peeled and cubed

Fresh chives, chopped, for garnish

1. Heat a braising pan (or a large, oven-safe skillet with a cover) over medium-high heat. Once the pan is hot, add the oil. Then add the lentils and garlic. Stir together for 1 minute.

2. Add the vegetable stock and bay leaf to the braising pan. Bring to a boil. Then add the thyme and tomato paste, using the back of a spoon to dissolve the paste into the stock.

3. Reduce the heat to medium, cover, and cook for about 15 minutes, stirring occasionally.

4. Remove the bay leaf.

5. In a small bowl, whisk together the tapioca flour and distilled water, then stir the mixture into the pan. (This will turn your broth into a thick gravy.)

6. Bring the ingredients in the braising pan to a simmer, then stir in the mixed vegetables, salt, and pepper.

7. Put the potatoes in a large saucepot filled half-way with water. Bring to a boil. Then reduce the heat to medium-high and cook until fork tender, about 20 minutes.

8. Preheat the oven to 350°F.

9. Drain the potatoes and mash them with a ricer, hand mixer, or fork.

10. Spread the mashed potatoes on top of the lentil mixture in the braising pan. Put the braising pan in the oven and bake for 25 minutes.

11. Just before serving, drizzle with olive oil and garnish with fresh chives.

~~~~~~

TIP: This is a great make-ahead dish. Spread the mashed potatoes on top of the lentil mixture and refrigerate until you are ready to bake and serve. You can also put it in individual sealed containers to be warmed and enjoyed during the week.

Farro and Vegetable Sauté

MAKE-AHEAD

SERVES 4 · PREP TIME: 20 MINUTES
COOK TIME: 35 TO 60 MINUTES, DEPENDING ON FARRO TYPE

This is a great make-ahead dish during your meal prep day. It has all of my favorite veggies in one place, but feel free to add other seasonal vegetables like sweet potatoes or butternut squash. Sometimes I top it with mint leaves or other fresh herbs I have handy.

2 cups uncooked farro
2 tablespoons coconut oil
½ cup finely chopped
   yellow onion
1 carrot, finely chopped
1 garlic clove, minced
6 ounces fresh green
   beans, chopped
1 summer squash, chopped
1 red or orange bell
   pepper, chopped
1 cup low-sodium
   vegetable broth
3 tablespoons
   tomato paste
1 cup frozen peas
1 teaspoon dried basil
½ teaspoon kosher salt
¼ teaspoon freshly ground
   black pepper
Fresh parsley, for garnish

1. Cook the farro according to the package instructions.

2. Heat the oil in a Dutch oven or large stockpot over medium heat. Sauté the onion and carrot for 1 minute. Then add the garlic and sauté for an additional 1 minute.

3. Add the green beans, summer squash, and bell pepper to the pan. Stir vigorously. Cook for 7 minutes.

4. In a small bowl, whisk together the vegetable broth and tomato paste, then pour the mixture into the pot with the vegetables.

5. Add the peas, basil, salt, and pepper. Stir to combine.

6. Bring the ingredients in the pot to a simmer. Cover and simmer for 5 minutes.

7. Add the farro to the ingredients in the pot. Stir together until warmed through, about 2 minutes.

8. Serve garnished with fresh parsley.

Quinoa-Vegetable Stew

30-MINUTE MEAL, ONE-POT

SERVES 4 BOWLS · PREP TIME: 20 MINUTES · COOK TIME: 25 MINUTES

Here's another one-pot wonder you're sure to love. Grab your Dutch oven and get your quinoa ready for a vegetable soirée. Garnish with fresh parsley or cilantro to bring all of the flavors together.

1 tablespoon coconut oil or olive oil
1 medium onion, chopped
1 red bell pepper, thinly sliced
3 garlic cloves, finely chopped
1 tablespoon paprika
1 teaspoon ground cumin
1 teaspoon kosher salt
½ teaspoon freshly ground black pepper
6 cups vegetable broth, plus more as needed
1 cup uncooked quinoa, rinsed
2 Roma tomatoes, coarsely chopped
1 cup frozen corn
1 cup frozen peas
1 avocado, halved, pitted and sliced
Fresh parsley or cilantro, chopped, for garnish

1. Heat the oil in a Dutch oven or large stockpot over medium heat. Add the onion and bell pepper, and sauté for 5 minutes.

2. Add the garlic, paprika, cumin, salt, and pepper. Stir together and let cook for about 1 minute.

3. Add the vegetable broth and bring to a boil.

4. Reduce the heat to medium and add the quinoa. Cook for 10 to 12 minutes.

5. Add the tomatoes, corn, and peas. Cook for another 5 to 7 minutes.

6. Serve topped with the avocado slices and garnished with fresh parsley or cilantro.

This is my comfort in my affliction, that your promise gives me life.
PSALM 119:50 (ESV)

Whatever affliction looks like, rest in His life-giving promises today knowing the eternal victory that you have because of Christ.

Fava Bean and Mushroom "Pot Roast"

FREEZER-FRIENDLY, MAKE-AHEAD

SERVES 4 • PREP TIME: 20 MINUTES • COOK TIME: 25 MINUTES

This is a great comfort food dish. With its rich, savory flavor and nutritious ingredients, it's sure to become a family favorite. You won't even miss the meat!

1 tablespoon olive oil
½ pound baby
   potatoes, halved
4 large portabella
   mushrooms, sliced into
   ¾-inch pieces
1 medium onion, chopped
2 large carrots, cut into
   3-inch pieces
2 garlic cloves, finely
   chopped
1 teaspoon dried thyme
1 teaspoon dried basil
1 teaspoon dried rosemary
1 teaspoon kosher salt
½ teaspoon freshly ground
   black pepper
3 cups vegetable broth
2 tablespoons
   tomato paste
¼ cup tapioca flour
¼ cup distilled water
1 (15-ounce) can fava
   beans, drained
   and rinsed

1. Heat the oil in a Dutch oven or large stockpot over medium heat. Add the potatoes and sauté for 7 minutes. Then add the mushrooms, onion, carrots, and garlic. Sauté for another 7 minutes, stirring occasionally.

2. Season with the thyme, basil, rosemary, salt, and pepper. Add the vegetable broth and tomato paste. Stir to combine. Bring to a simmer.

3. In a small bowl, whisk together the tapioca flour and distilled water. Stir the mixture into the pot. (This will thicken up your sauce.)

4. Stir in the fava beans, cover, and cook for another 10 to 13 minutes, or until the potatoes are fork-tender.

5. Ladle the "pot roast" into bowls or serve family style.

TIP: This dish can also be prepared in your slow cooker on medium heat during the day. Just add all the ingredients except for the tapioca flour mixture and fava beans. When you get home, increase the temperature to high, stir in the tapioca flour mixture and beans, and let cook for 15 minutes.

Lemon-Artichoke Zucchini Noodles

30-MINUTE MEAL

SERVES 4 • PREP TIME: 20 MINUTES • COOK TIME: 5 MINUTES

Here's the Italian in me again! These flavors together say you're in Tuscany enjoying a delicious pasta dish while sitting outside and enjoying the view. The zucchini noodles absorb the lemon flavor so deliciously that you won't miss the pasta.

5 to 6 medium zucchini

1½ teaspoons kosher
    salt, divided

2 tablespoons coconut oil
    or olive oil

1 can quartered
    artichokes, drained

2 garlic cloves,
    finely chopped

¼ cup capers, drained

½ teaspoon freshly ground
    black pepper

1 tablespoon freshly
    squeezed lemon juice

½ cup chopped fresh
    parsley or fresh basil

1. Cut the ends off the zucchini and turn them into ribbons, either by using a spiralizer on the ribbon setting or by using a vegetable peeler. Season the zucchini noodles with 1 teaspoon of salt and put them in a colander covered with a paper towel for 20 minutes. (This removes the moisture.)

2. Heat the oil in a large sauté pan over medium-high heat. Add the artichokes and garlic. Cook for 30 seconds. Then add the zucchini noodles. Using tongs, toss to combine the ingredients for 1 minute.

3. Add the capers, the remaining ½ teaspoon salt, and the pepper. Continue tossing while cooking for another minute or two.

4. Remove the pan from the heat and transfer the contents to a large serving bowl. Toss in the lemon juice and fresh herbs, and serve!

Roasted Chiles Rellenos with Cashew Cheese

SERVES 4 · PREP TIME: 20 MINUTES, PLUS 2 HOURS TO SOAK THE CASHEWS
COOK TIME: 50 MINUTES

Break out the cast-iron pan for this one! Between the roasted peppers stuffed with beans and the melted cashew cheese, this is a Daniel Fast fiesta!

1 cup raw cashews
¼ cup distilled water
½ teaspoon cumin
¼ teaspoon sea salt
¼ teaspoon garlic powder
¼ teaspoon chili powder
4 poblano peppers, whole
1 tablespoon extra-virgin
   olive oil
1 small onion, chopped
2 garlic cloves, minced
2 jalapeño peppers, sliced
1 red bell pepper, chopped
1 can diced tomatoes
   with chiles
½ teaspoon kosher salt
½ teaspoon freshly ground
   black pepper
½ cup vegetable stock or
   distilled water
1 teaspoon dried oregano
1 teaspoon chili powder
1 teaspoon coriander
1 teaspoon cumin
1 (15-ounce) can black
   beans, drained
   and rinsed
Fresh cilantro, chopped,
   for garnish

1. Soak the cashews in water for a minimum of 2 hours.

2. To make the cashew cheese, drain the cashews and put them in a blender with the distilled water, cumin, sea salt, garlic powder, and chili powder. Blend until smooth, transfer to a bowl, and cover.

3. Preheat the oven to 400°F. Line a baking sheet with parchment paper.

4. Slice the poblano peppers down the center, leaving the stem in place. (This is where you'll add the stuffing later on.) Roast them on the baking sheet for 10 minutes, then take them out and set them aside. Leave the oven on.

5. Heat the olive oil in a cast-iron pan over medium heat. Sauté the onion, garlic, jalapeño peppers, and bell pepper for 5 minutes, stirring occasionally.

6. Stir in the diced tomatoes with chiles, and season with kosher salt and pepper. Let cook for another 5 minutes.

7. Add the vegetable stock, followed by the oregano, chili powder, coriander, and cumin. Stir to combine. Cook for 5 minutes, or until the liquid is reduced by half.

8. In a small bowl, use a fork to *lightly* mash the black beans. (Don't smooth the beans to a puree. Keep them chunky.)

9. Take ¼ cup of the sauce mixture from the pan, add it to the beans, and stir to combine.

10. Fill each roasted poblano pepper with some bean mixture, some sauce from the pan, and some cashew cheese. Then place the peppers in the cast-iron pan on top of the sauce mixture and top with any remaining cashew cheese.

11. Cover the cast-iron pan with foil and bake for 20 minutes. Uncover the pan and bake for an additional 5 minutes. Top with cilantro and enjoy!

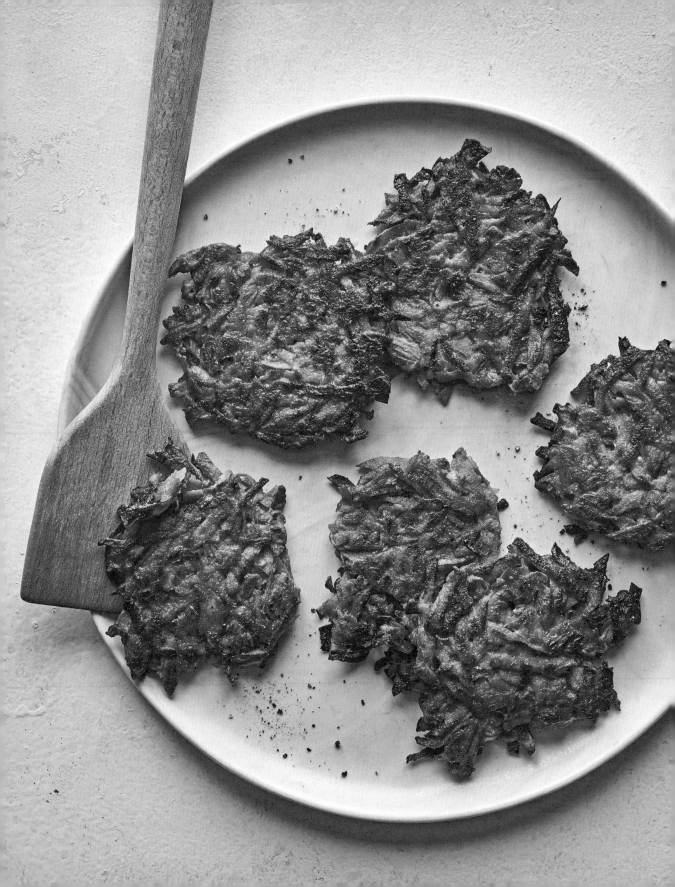

CHAPTER 9

Sides and Snacks

< Sweet Potato Latkes

Roasted Mushrooms

SERVES 4 • PREP TIME: 10 MINUTES • COOK TIME: 20 MINUTES

Every great dish deserves something on the side to bring the flavors all together. This one is made to be versatile. Serve these mushrooms warm with your family dinners, cool with a green salad, or on their own as a hearty appetizer. Any mushrooms will work, but I recommend bella mushrooms, which keep their texture well when roasted.

2 pounds whole mushrooms
2 tablespoons extra-virgin olive oil
1½ teaspoons garlic powder
1 teaspoon dried thyme
1 teaspoon kosher salt
½ teaspoon freshly ground black pepper
½ teaspoon dried parsley
Balsamic vinegar
Fresh herbs, for garnish

1. Put the oven rack in the center position. Preheat the oven to 400°F. Line a large baking sheet with parchment paper.

2. Put the mushrooms in a large bowl. Add the olive oil, garlic powder, thyme, salt, pepper, and dried parsley. Stir well to combine.

3. Spread the mushrooms in an even layer on the prepared baking sheet and roast for 20 minutes, or until tender, flipping the mushrooms over halfway through.

4. Drizzle with balsamic vinegar before serving, and garnish with fresh herbs.

TIP: Mushrooms from the grocery store will stay fresh for about 2 days. To increase their lifetime by a few days, remove the mushrooms from their package and put them in an airtight container with a paper towel at the bottom.

Zucchini Chips

SERVES 2 • PREP TIME: 15 MINUTES • COOK TIME: 2 HOURS

Craving a snack? These Zucchini Chips are the perfect Daniel Fast–approved snack that everyone will enjoy! Be sure to flip after the first hour to ensure a crisp bite on both sides.

1 large zucchini
2 to 3 tablespoons
    extra-virgin olive oil
1 to 1½ teaspoons sea salt

1. Preheat the oven to 225°F. Line two large baking sheets with parchment paper.

2. Slice the zucchini into very thin rounds using a chef's knife or mandoline.

3. Line your countertop or another large, clean work surface with paper towels. Lay the sliced zucchini out on the paper towels in an even layer. Then top with another paper towel and lightly press. Let rest for 10 minutes.

4. Spread the zucchini slices in an even layer on the prepared baking sheets and brush the tops lightly with oil.

5. Bake for 1 hour, then flip the zucchini over and brush the other side with oil. Bake for another hour, or until golden and starting to crisp.

6. Lightly season with salt and serve, or store in an airtight container for up to 2 days.

Roasted Vegetable Medley

SERVES 4 · PREP TIME: 15 MINUTES · COOK TIME: 20 MINUTES

This side dish will easily steal the show with colorful and hearty ingredients like peppers, broccoli, and onions. Add the potatoes to the vegetables just before serving and give them a quick toss in some olive oil for added freshness.

1 pound small yellow potatoes, whole
3 tablespoons olive oil, divided
1 red bell pepper, sliced
1 medium zucchini, sliced
1 head broccoli, cut into florets
1 (8-ounce) package mushrooms, whole (any kind)
1 medium red onion, sliced
1 teaspoon Italian seasoning
1 teaspoon garlic powder
1 teaspoon onion powder
1 teaspoon dried oregano
1 teaspoon dried parsley
1 teaspoon kosher salt
½ teaspoon freshly ground black pepper
Fresh parsley, for garnish

1. Preheat the oven to 400°F. Line two baking sheets with parchment paper.

2. Put the potatoes in a large bowl and drizzle with 1 tablespoon olive oil. Then stir to coat. Spread the potatoes in an even layer on one of the prepared baking sheets and roast for 40 minutes, or until fork-tender.

3. Put the bell pepper, zucchini, broccoli florets, mushrooms, and red onion on the other baking sheet. Roast for 20 to 25 minutes.

4. Transfer the vegetables (not the potatoes) to a large bowl. Drizzle with 1 tablespoon olive oil. Then add the Italian seasoning, garlic powder, onion powder, oregano, parsley, salt, and pepper. Stir to coat.

5. Add the potatoes and stir to combine with the vegetables.

6. Serve on a platter drizzled with the remaining 1 tablespoon of oil and garnished with the fresh parsley.

The thief comes only to steal and kill and destroy. I have come that they may have life, and have it to the full.

JOHN 10:10

In this parable, Christ is demonstrating His role as the Good Shepherd. Those who do not know Him will not follow His voice because they do not follow the voice of strangers. Seek His voice today, and rest in the promise that in Him you will have everything you need.

Sweet Potato Latkes

FREEZER-FRIENDLY

SERVES 4 · PREP TIME: 20 MINUTES · COOK TIME: 15 MINUTES

Planning ahead for snack attacks is crucial when following any dietary restrictions, so a freezer- and family-friendly bite is a necessity! My family loves these Sweet Potato Latkes so much that we always make double batches. The key is frying small, uncrowded batches of latkes in a very hot pan.

2 tablespoons
flaxseed meal

5 tablespoons
distilled water

1 pound sweet potatoes,
peeled and grated

⅓ cup chickpea flour

1 teaspoon kosher salt

½ teaspoon freshly ground
black pepper

Coconut oil or olive oil,
for frying

1. To make flax eggs, whisk together the flaxseed meal and distilled water in a small bowl. Let the mixture sit for 5 to 15 minutes.

2. In a large mixing bowl, combine the sweet potatoes, chickpea flour, flax eggs, salt, and pepper.

3. Heat a large, deep skillet or cast-iron pan over medium-high heat. When the pan is hot, add about 2 tablespoons of oil. Let the oil get very hot.

4. Place a few heaping tablespoons of the sweet potato mixture in the pan, evenly spaced, and fry for 3 minutes. Then flip and fry the latkes for another 2 to 3 minutes, until golden brown. Transfer them to a large platter lined with paper towels.

5. Continue cooking the latkes in small batches—don't overcrowd the pan—until you've used all the sweet potato mixture. Enjoy!

TIP: Store these latkes in a sealable container or bag in the refrigerator for up to 5 days or in the freezer for up to 2 months.

Roasted Acorn Squash with Kale and Pecans

SERVES 2 · PREP TIME: 15 MINUTES · COOK TIME: 35 MINUTES

The toasted pecans that top this dish are like the toppings on a sundae! It's a delicious way to warm up on a cold winter's night. Lay the slices of acorn squash on a platter and surround them with sautéed kale for a presentation that'll wow your guests.

1 acorn squash
3 tablespoons extra-virgin olive oil, divided
1 large bunch of kale, chopped
2 garlic cloves, minced
1 shallot, finely chopped
1 teaspoon kosher salt
½ teaspoon freshly ground black pepper
¼ cup raw pecans

1. Preheat the oven to 400°F. Line a large baking sheet with parchment paper.

2. Cut the acorn squash in half, remove the seeds, and chop into 1-inch pieces. (Keep the skin on—it's edible when cooked!)

3. Lay the squash pieces in an even layer on the baking sheet and drizzle with 2 tablespoons of olive oil. Roast for 20 to 25 minutes or until fork-tender.

4. Heat 1 tablespoon of olive oil in a large sauté pan over medium heat. Add the kale and sauté, tossing with tongs, for 2 minutes. Add the garlic, shallot, salt, and pepper, and cook for another 5 minutes.

5. Take the squash pieces and lay them on a large platter. Place the kale around the squash pieces.

6. Heat the sauté pan over medium heat. Add the pecans and toast for about 1 minute, stirring vigorously to make sure all sides of the pecans are toasted.

7. Sprinkle the pecans over the squash and kale, and serve.

White Bean Hummus

SERVES 4 • PREP TIME: 5 MINUTES

If company is on the way, this "hummus" is the ideal quick fix. It pairs perfectly with carrot sticks, cucumbers, or even celery sticks. For even more options for your guests, add a bowl of Creamy Dill Sauce (page 150).

1 (15-ounce) can cannellini beans, drained and rinsed

2 tablespoons all-natural tahini (100% sesame seeds)

2 tablespoons extra-virgin olive oil

Juice of 1 lemon

1 garlic clove, peeled

½ teaspoon sea salt

1. Put the cannellini beans, tahini, olive oil, lemon juice, garlic, and salt in a blender or food processor. Blend until smooth.

2. If the hummus is too thick, add more olive oil 1 teaspoon at a time while blending. Serve in a bowl.

TIP: Try replacing the tahini with sesame oil and adding ¾ teaspoon of cumin.

5-Layer Guacamole Dip

SERVES 4 · PREP TIME: 10 MINUTES

Who doesn't love a layered dip? The key here is the freshness of the homemade guacamole, bursting with hints of lime, chili powder, and garlic. Once your dip is assembled, it'll look too good to eat—almost. Since chips are off-limits during the Daniel Fast, I love serving this dip with a variety of vegetables.

2 to 3 fresh avocados, halved and pitted

Juice of 1 lime

½ teaspoon cumin

½ teaspoon chili powder

½ teaspoon garlic powder

½ teaspoon sea salt, plus more

1 (16-ounce) can vegetarian refried beans

2 cups all-natural salsa, mild or hot

1 bell pepper, chopped

½ cup black olives, halved

3 scallions, thinly sliced

2 Roma tomatoes, diced

1. Scoop the avocado flesh into a bowl and mash it with a fork. Mix in the lime juice, cumin, chili powder, garlic powder, and sea salt. This is your guacamole.

2. To create your layers, start by lining the bottom of an 8-by-8-inch glass baking dish with the refried beans. Then create a layer of salsa, followed by a layer of guacamole, followed by a layer of bell pepper, black olives, and scallions. Finish it off with a layer of diced tomato.

So do not fear, for I am with you; do not be dismayed, for I am your God. I will strengthen you and help you; I will uphold you with my righteous right hand.

ISAIAH 41:10

Whatever this day holds—the fears you have, the circumstances you're facing, that one problem that won't go away—remember that the Lord will strengthen you and give you the grace you need to take one step at a time.

Buffalo Cauliflower Dip

SERVES 4 · PREP TIME: 15 MINUTES, PLUS 2 HOURS TO SOAK THE CASHEWS
COOK TIME: 40 MINUTES

Here's another mouthwatering reason to soak your cashews! Take your roasted cauliflower to the food processor and blend it with the flavors of your favorite all-natural hot sauce and some fresh garlic. Serve hot with fresh vegetable slices for a distinctly un-guilty pleasure.

1 cup raw cashews
1 head cauliflower, chopped into florets
1 (15-ounce) can chickpeas, drained and rinsed
1 garlic clove, chopped
¾ cup all-natural hot sauce
Juice of 1 lemon
½ teaspoon kosher salt
½ teaspoon paprika
¼ to ½ cup distilled water, room temperature
2 to 3 scallions, thinly sliced

1. Soak the raw cashews in water for at least 2 hours.

2. Preheat the oven to 400°F. Line a baking sheet with parchment paper.

3. Spread the cauliflower florets in an even layer on the baking sheet. Roast for 20 minutes. Remove the cauliflower from the oven and reduce the oven's temperature to 350°F.

4. Drain the soaked cashews and put them in a blender or food processor with the roasted cauliflower florets, chickpeas, garlic, hot sauce, lemon juice, salt, and paprika. Pulse a few times, slowly add some of the distilled water, and pulse a few more times. Continue until you have a thick sauce with small chunks of cauliflower.

5. Pour the dip into a large ramekin or oven-safe bowl and bake at 350°F for 20 minutes.

6. Top with scallions and serve with fresh vegetable slices.

~~~~~~

TIP: You can also use frozen cauliflower florets instead of fresh—no adjustments to the recipe needed.

Vegetarian Fried Cauliflower Rice

SERVES 4 · PREP TIME: 15 TO 30 MINUTES · COOK TIME: 15 MINUTES

Make mealtime even easier with frozen vegetables in this quick and easy dish. In just 15 minutes, this flavor-packed cauliflower rice will be ready to eat as a side dish (or even a meal). You'll love the protein and veggies in every bite.

1 pound firm tofu
2 tablespoons olive oil or sesame oil
1 head cauliflower, riced
1 garlic clove, minced
½-inch piece fresh ginger, peeled and grated
1 cup frozen carrots, thawed
1 cup frozen petite peas, thawed
1 cup frozen corn, thawed
2 to 3 scallions, sliced, divided

1. To prepare the tofu, lay a few paper towels on a plate or other clean work surface. Set the tofu on top. Then put several more paper towels on top of the tofu. Place a heavy pan or other heavy item on top of the paper towels and let them sit for 10 to 30 minutes. (This presses the moisture out of the tofu.) When you're done pressing out the moisture, cut the tofu into ½-inch cubes.

2. Heat a large skillet or wok over medium-high heat. Once the pan is hot, add the oil and let it get hot.

3. Add the tofu, sautéing each side for about 3 minutes. Add the cauliflower, garlic, and ginger, and sauté for an additional 5 minutes, stirring occasionally.

4. Stir in the carrots, peas, and corn. Cook for 5 to 7 minutes. Stir in half the scallions and remove the pan from the heat.

5. Serve garnished with the remaining scallions.

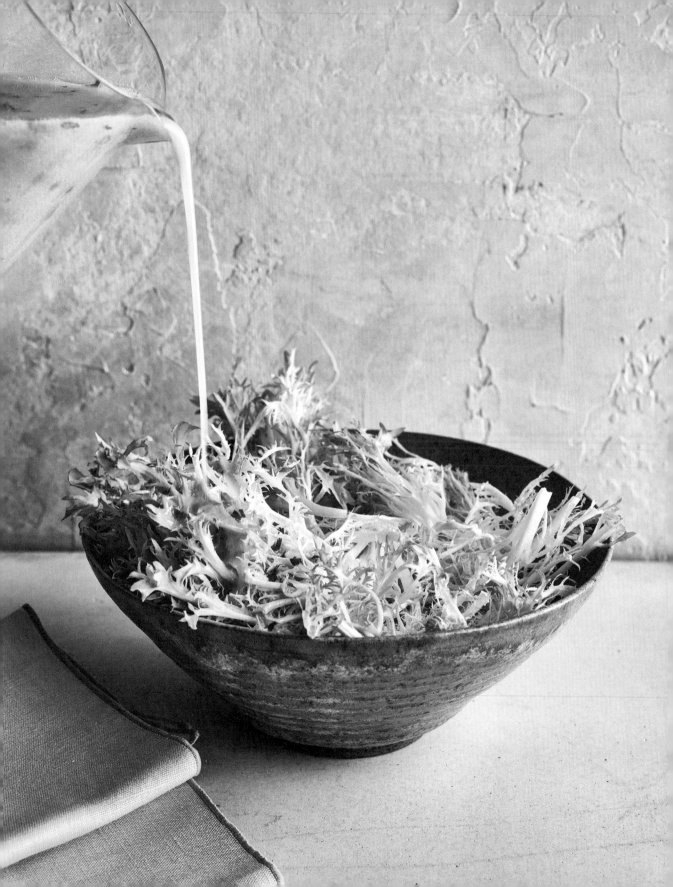

CHAPTER 10

Sauces and Dressings

< Dijon Vinaigrette

Green Goodness Dressing

MAKES ¾ CUP • PREP TIME: 10 MINUTES

This creamy and delicious dressing is my vegan and Daniel Fast–friendly take on "green goddess" dressing! It goes well in many of the recipes in this book and makes a perfect dip for crudités or lettuce wraps. Feel free to add more of any of the flavors, or include other fresh herbs such as tarragon and chives.

2 small avocados, peeled and pitted
1 cup packed basil leaves
2 tablespoons apple cider vinegar
2 scallions, chopped
Juice of 1 lemon
1 garlic clove, chopped
1 teaspoon kosher salt
½ teaspoon freshly ground black pepper
½ cup avocado oil

1. Put the avocado, basil leaves, apple cider vinegar, scallions, lemon juice, garlic, salt, and pepper in a food processor or blender.

2. Blend the ingredients. While the blender is on, drizzle in the avocado oil until the mixture becomes smooth. (If the mixture becomes too thick, add in water 1 teaspoon at a time until it reaches the consistency of salad dressing.)

Pesto with Walnuts

FREEZER-FRIENDLY, MAKE-AHEAD

MAKES ½ CUP • PREP TIME: 10 MINUTES

The simple ingredients in pesto brighten any dish, and it's perfect for storing to use later. Keep it in a sealed plastic container in the refrigerator for up to a week or the freezer for up to 3 months. Adding some lemon juice will help it keep that vibrant green color.

2 cups firmly packed fresh basil
¼ cup extra-virgin olive oil
2 tablespoons walnuts, chopped
1 garlic clove, roughly chopped
½ teaspoon kosher salt

Put all the ingredients in a blender or food processor, and process until smooth.

Creamy Dill Sauce

MAKES 1½ CUP • PREP TIME: 10 MINUTES, PLUS 2 HOURS FOR THE CASHEWS TO SOAK

This easy dill sauce is hearty and full of flavor. The soaked cashews provide a creamy, filling base for the sauce (and plenty of protein).

1 cup raw cashews
½ cup distilled water
¾ cup chopped fresh dill
1 tablespoon freshly
   squeezed lemon juice
1 teaspoon chopped
   shallot
1 garlic clove, chopped
1 teaspoon kosher salt
½ teaspoon freshly ground
   black pepper
½ cup extra-virgin olive oil

1. Soak the cashews in the water for a minimum of 2 hours. Drain them and put them in a blender.

2. Add the dill, lemon juice, shallot, garlic, salt, and pepper to the blender. Start to blend, slowly drizzling in the olive oil until the mixture reaches a thick and creamy consistency.

Jesus looked at them and said, "With man this is impossible, but not with God; all things are possible with God."

MARK 10:27

So many times I find myself trying to put God in a box. However, what looks impossible to us gives us a glimpse at the power of our Creator. Rest in this promise today.

Homestyle Italian Herb Dressing

MAKE-AHEAD

MAKES ¾ CUP • PREP TIME: 10 MINUTES

During the Daniel Fast, I like to keep the recipes simple yet full of flavor. I believe this dressing will add the perfect pop of flavor to your salads and bowls.

¾ cup extra-virgin olive oil
½ cup apple cider vinegar
1 garlic clove, minced
1 teaspoon minced shallot
1 teaspoon dried oregano
1 teaspoon dried basil
½ teaspoon dried thyme
½ teaspoon kosher salt
¼ teaspoon freshly ground
  black pepper

Put all the ingredients in a canning jar. Cover and shake.

TIP: This is a great make-ahead dressing that will last all week in your refrigerator. Be sure to take it out 30 minutes before using and shake it well just before adding it to your salad.

Dijon Vinaigrette

MAKES 1 CUP • PREP TIME: 10 MINUTES

The creamy texture and flavor Dijon mustard gives to this vinaigrette is perfect for your salads, bowls, and even main dishes. I love to cut up fresh vegetables and dip them in this dressing as a snack.

⅓ cup apple cider vinegar
4 basil leaves
1 tablespoon Dijon mustard
1 garlic clove, peeled
1 teaspoon fresh parsley
¼ teaspoon kosher salt
¼ teaspoon freshly ground black pepper
¾ cup extra-virgin olive oil

1. Put the vinegar, basil, Dijon mustard, garlic, parsley, salt, and pepper in a blender.

2. Start to blend, slowly drizzling in the olive oil until the dressing reaches a smooth consistency.

TIP: You can store this dressing in a canning jar or other covered container in your refrigerator for up to a week. Just shake and enjoy over your salad for lunch!

Caper Vinaigrette

MAKES ½ CUP • PREP TIME: 10 MINUTES

This dressing pairs robust flavors from the spice rack with lemon zest and capers, giving you the perfect balance for a vinaigrette that everyone can enjoy—even the folks who generally prefer Thousand Island.

3 tablespoons finely chopped fresh parsley

2 tablespoons capers, drained and finely chopped

1 garlic clove, minced

1 shallot, finely chopped

1 tablespoon freshly squeezed lemon juice

Zest of 1 lemon

½ teaspoon kosher salt

¼ teaspoon freshly ground black pepper

½ cup extra-virgin olive oil

1. In a small bowl, whisk together the parsley, capers, garlic, shallot, lemon juice, lemon zest, salt, and pepper.

2. Continue whisking while gradually pouring in extra-virgin olive oil until the dressing reaches your desired consistency.

Simple Marinara Sauce

FREEZER-FRIENDLY

MAKES 6 CUPS • PREP TIME: 10 MINUTES • COOK TIME: 35 MINUTES

Every Sunday my Nana would have a big pot of marinara simmering for the entire day. We'd all stand by the stove and dip bread in it. By the time we ate dinner, the loaf was gone. I still make a big pot of marinara on a regular basis and freeze some for later!

⅓ cup olive oil
½ cup finely diced yellow onion
2 garlic cloves, minced
¼ teaspoon red pepper flakes
4 cups canned San Marzano Italian plum tomatoes in their juices
1 (7-ounce) can organic tomato paste
2 teaspoons dried basil
1½ teaspoons kosher salt
1 teaspoon freshly ground black pepper
1 teaspoon dried oregano
1 teaspoon dried parsley
½ teaspoon dried thyme

1. Heat the olive oil in a large pot over medium-high heat. Add the onion and sauté for 30 seconds. Reduce the heat to medium. Add the garlic and red pepper flakes, and sauté for an additional 30 seconds.

2. Add the tomatoes to the pot and bring to a boil. Using a teaspoon, add the tomato paste to the pot by pressing the paste against the edge of the pot. To get any remaining tomato paste out of the can, fill the can with hot water, stir it with the teaspoon, and pour it into the pot.

3. Add the basil, salt, pepper, oregano, parsley, and thyme to the pot, stirring to combine.

4. Bring the ingredients in the pot to a boil. Cover and reduce the heat to a simmer. Simmer for 15 to 30 minutes.

TIP: Divide up any unused sauce into sealable 16-ounce plastic freezer bags. They stack nicely and don't take up a lot of room in the freezer. Each bag holds about 2 cups, which is perfect to feed two people.

Cashew Gravy

FREEZER-FRIENDLY

MAKES 2 CUPS · PREP TIME: 5 MINUTES · COOK TIME: 7 MINUTES

This is a great sauce to use if you're having friends over who are curious about your new fast and what it means for the dinner table. This recipe proves that gravy can be exciting to taste and easy to make, even when it's plant-based.

2 cups low-sodium vegetable broth or distilled water
½ cup raw, unsalted cashews
2 tablespoons arrowroot flour
1 garlic clove, peeled
1 teaspoon onion powder
½ teaspoon kosher salt
½ teaspoon freshly ground black pepper

1. In a blender, blend the broth, cashews, arrowroot flour, garlic, onion powder, and salt until smooth.

2. Pour into a small saucepan over medium heat and whisk continuously until it reaches a gravy-like consistency, about 7 minutes. (If it becomes too thick, add 1 more tablespoon of water or vegetable broth.)

3. Season with the black pepper before serving.

TIP: Freeze any unused gravy in a sealable plastic bag or container. To reheat, warm in a saucepan over medium-low heat for about 5 minutes, whisking continuously. Add a tablespoon of water or vegetable broth if the consistency becomes too thick.

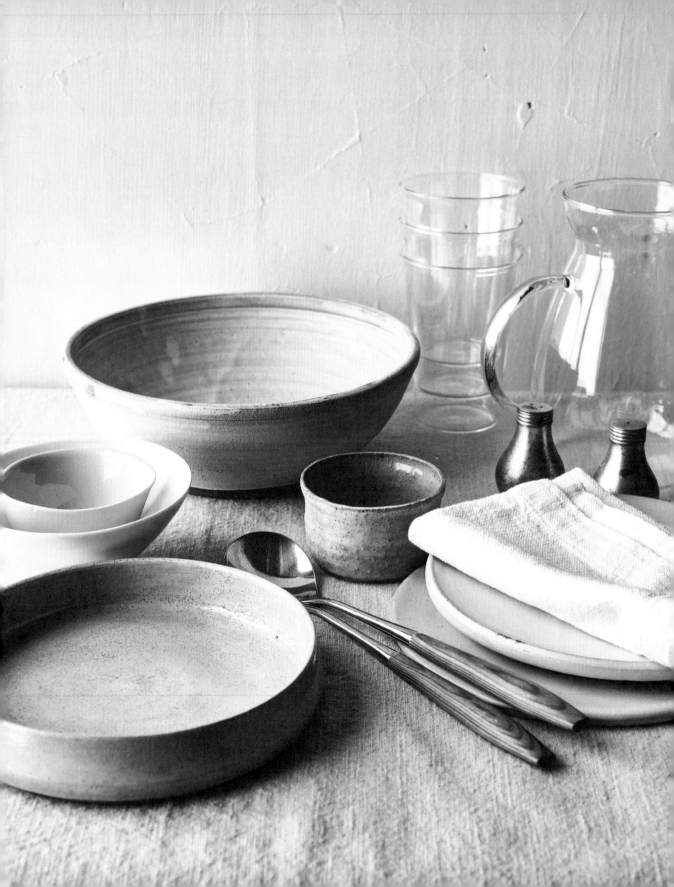

Measurement Conversions

	US STANDARD	US STANDARD (OUNCES)	METRIC (APPROXIMATE)
VOLUME EQUIVALENTS (LIQUID)	2 tablespoons	1 fl. oz.	30 mL
	¼ cup	2 fl. oz.	60 mL
	½ cup	4 fl. oz.	120 mL
	1 cup	8 fl. oz.	240 mL
	1½ cups	12 fl. oz.	355 mL
	2 cups or 1 pint	16 fl. oz.	475 mL
	4 cups or 1 quart	32 fl. oz.	1 L
	1 gallon	128 fl. oz.	4 L
VOLUME EQUIVALENTS (DRY)	⅛ teaspoon		0.5 mL
	¼ teaspoon		1 mL
	½ teaspoon		2 mL
	¾ teaspoon		4 mL
	1 teaspoon		5 mL
	1 tablespoon		15 mL
	¼ cup		59 mL
	⅓ cup		79 mL
	½ cup		118 mL
	⅔ cup		156 mL
	¾ cup		177 mL
	1 cup		235 mL
	2 cups or 1 pint		475 mL
	3 cups		700 mL
	4 cups or 1 quart		1 L
	½ gallon		2 L
	1 gallon		4 L
WEIGHT EQUIVALENTS	½ ounce		15 g
	1 ounce		30 g
	2 ounces		60 g
	4 ounces		115 g
	8 ounces		225 g
	12 ounces		340 g
	16 ounces or 1 pound		455 g

	FAHRENHEIT (F)	CELSIUS (C) (APPROXIMATE)
OVEN TEMPERATURES	250°F	120°C
	300°F	150°C
	325°F	180°C
	375°F	190°C
	400°F	200°C
	425°F	220°C
	450°F	230°C

References

Centers for Disease Control and Prevention. "What Noises Cause Hearing Loss?" Last modified October 7, 2019. https://cdc.gov/nceh/hearing_loss/what _noises_cause_hearing_loss.html.

Craig, Winston J. "Health Effects of Vegan Diets." *The American Journal of Clinical Nutrition* 89, no. 5 (May 2009): 1627S–1633S. https://doi.org/10.3945 /ajcn.2009.26736N.

Damico, Matt. "The World Needs You to Be Different." Desiring God. Last modified March 5, 2017. https://www.desiringgod.org/articles/the-world -needs-you-to-be-different.

Greear, J. D. *Gospel: Recovering the Power That Made Christianity Revolutionary*. Nashville: B&H Publishing Group, 2011.

Kahleova, Hana, Susan Levin, and Neal Barnard. "Cardio-Metabolic Benefits of Plant-Based Diets," in "The Science of Vegetarian Nutrition and Health," ed. Karen Jaceldo-Siegl, special issue, *Nutrients* 9, no. 8 (2017): 848. https://doi .org/10.3390/nu9080848.

Kerr, Gordon. "Soy Protein Vs. Meat Protein." Livestrong.com. Last modified February 21, 2019. https://www.livestrong.com/article/240951-soy-protein-vs -meat-protein/.

Liu, Rui Hai. "Health Benefits of Fruits and Vegetables Are from Additive and Synergistic Combinations of Phytochemicals." *The American Journal of Clinical Nutrition* 78, no. 3 (September 2003): 517S–520S. https://doi.org /10.1093/ajcn/78.3.517S.

Mathis, David. *Habits of Grace: Enjoying Jesus through the Spiritual Disciplines*. Nashville: Crossway, 2016.

Piper, John. "What Is the Purpose of Fasting?" Desiring God. Last modified April 18, 2013. https://www.desiringgod.org/interviews/what-is-the-purpose -of-fasting.

TerKeurst, Lysa. *Trustworthy: Overcoming Our Greatest Struggles to Trust God.* Nashville: LifeWay Press, 2019.

TerKeurst, Lysa. *Uninvited: Living Loved When You Feel Less Than, Left Out, and Lonely.* Nashville: Thomas Nelson, 2016.

Tuso, Phillip J., Mohamed H. Ismail, Benjamin P. Ha, and Carole Bartolotto. "Nutritional Update for Physicians: Plant-Based Diets." *The Permanente Journal* 17, no. 2 (spring 2013): 61–66. https://doi.org/10.7812/TPP/12-085.

Villines, Zawn. "Top 15 Sources of Plant-Based Protein Foods." Medical News Today. Last modified April 12, 2018. https://www.medicalnewstoday.com/articles/321474.

Whitney, Donald S. *Spiritual Disciplines for the Christian Life.* Colorado Springs: NavPress, 2014.

Zieliniski, Sarah. "Secrets of a Lion's Roar." SmithsonianMag.com. Last modified November 3, 2011. https://www.smithsonianmag.com/science-nature/secrets-of-a-lions-roar-126395997.

Index

C

Acknowledgments

The first person I need to thank and acknowledge is my husband, Glenn. You are always supportive of my endeavors and continue to encourage me on a daily basis.

To my daughter and son, Nikki and Steven, I love you both so very much! From the beginning, you have been my favorite people to cook for and share a meal with. My heart is so full of joy, pride, and gratitude when I think of you. I pray that Jesus will continue weaving his amazing God-story of grace over you and your families.

Kelly Stutle, thank you for your research in the Bible scriptures and devotionals. Your dedication was a true blessing.

Leia Vincent, your schedule is so busy, yet you still found time to give me advice on my recipes. I am extremely grateful to call you my daughter-in-law.

Thank you to my friends at Orange Theory. You've all been the best taste testers and cheered me on while working on this book.

Thank you to Christ Fellowship Church, my church family, and Pastors Todd and Julie Mullins, for sharing the hope and love of Jesus so I could experience it fully, in worship and in God's Word. I am so grateful to know I belong at the banquet table as a daughter of the King.

To the ladies in my sisterhood circle, I'm grateful for your bonds of friendship and how God used you to encourage me, teach me, and grow my faith. You opened my eyes so I could see God's purpose and gifts in me, and use them for God's family.

God also blessed me with two wonderful brothers in Christ, Dave Simiele and Kevin Wilson, without whom this book wouldn't have been possible. Thank you for your belief in me and for your amazing support as I learned how to serve God's family with you through ministry and team-building events.

And, of course, all glory to Jesus! I was lost, but Your invitation made all the difference. Thank You for saving me a seat at Your table.

About the Author

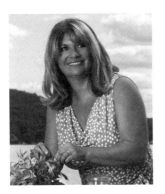

Cindy Anschutz is a chef, TV personality, entrepreneur, and true believer who fills her life with faith, family, and food. With more than 18 years of experience as a personal chef, Cindy has also appeared on cooking segments across local and national TV stations, connecting with families and sharing her recipes for a healthier, more flavorful lifestyle. Her previous cookbooks, *Cindy's Table* and *Paleo Italian Cooking*, showcase her love for Italian cooking around specific food sensitivities while maintaining an upscale yet approachable taste. She lives in Palm Beach Gardens, Florida, with her husband, Glenn, and their dog, Jake.